ESSENCE

TOTAL MAKEOVER
BODY, BEAUTY, SPIRIT

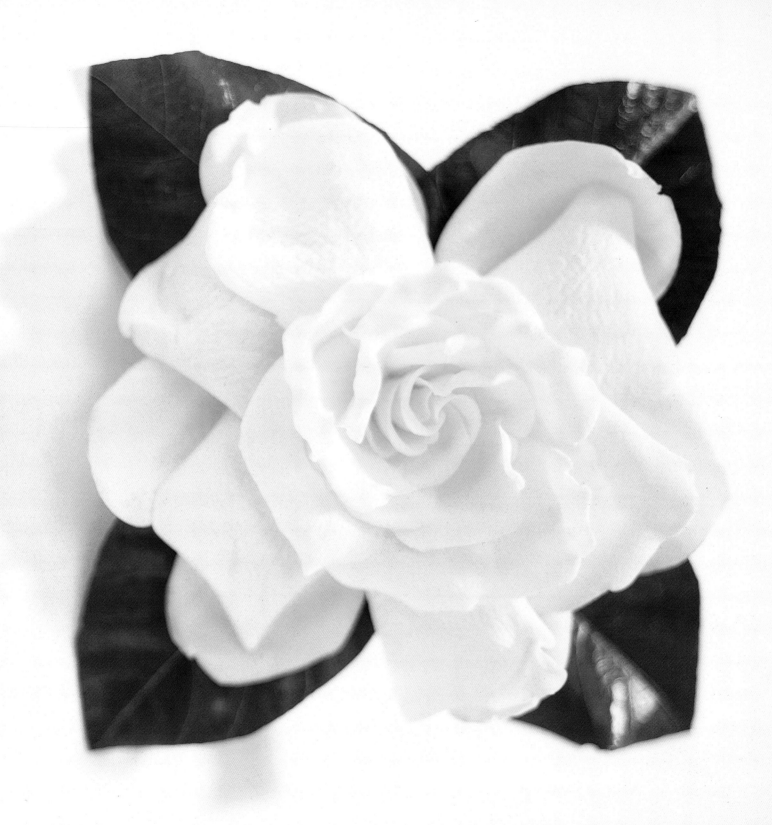

ESSENCE

TOTAL MAKEOVER
BODY, BEAUTY, SPIRIT

INTRODUCTION BY SUSAN L. TAYLOR

PATRICIA MIGNON HINDS, EDITOR

THREE RIVERS PRESS / NEW YORK

Published by Three Rivers Press, New York, New York.
Member of the Crown Publishing Group.

Random House, Inc. New York, Toronto, London, Sydney, Auckland
www.randomhouse.com

THREE RIVERS PRESS is a registered trademark and the Three Rivers Press colophon is a trademark of Random House, Inc.

Printed in China

Design by Elizabeth Van Itallie

Library of Congress Cataloging-in-Publication Data
The Essence Total Makeover: Body, Beauty, Spirit / Patricia Mignon Hinds, editor.
Includes bibliographical references.
1. Beauty, Personal. 2. African-American women. I. Essence.
RA778.4.A36E87   2000
646.7'042'08996073 dc21   99-14442

ISBN 0-609-80527-4

10 9 8 7 6 5 4 3

CONTRIBUTORS

Rachel Christmas Derrick

Angela Dodson

Tamala Edwards

Deborah Gregory

Pamela Johnson

Jenyne Raines

Tina L. Redwood

Tara Roberts

Knox Robinson

Teresa Wiltz

Tracy Harford, Photo Editor

ADVISORS

Linda Anderson, Ph.D.

John Atchison, John Atchison Hair Salons

Diane Bailey, Tendrils House of Ujamma

Beatrice Brown, Ph.D., BSB Wholistic Health Center

Constance Brown-Riggs, M.S.Ed.

Diane Dacosta, Dyaspora Hair Salon and Day Spa

Irma Denson, Irma Denson Skin Care Salon and Day Spa

Ryan Gentles, Zion Physical Wellness

Dr. Jennifer D. Harris

Sharone Huey, New York Sports Training Institute

Ziba Kashef

Ellin LaVar, LaVar Hair Designs

Dr. Reginald Manning

Werner Mendel, New Age Health Spa

Dr. Carlyle H. Miller

Dr. Luther K. Robinson

Jan Robinson, P.N.P.

Dr. Deborah A. Simmons

Wanda Wheeler, M.S.W.

CONTENTS

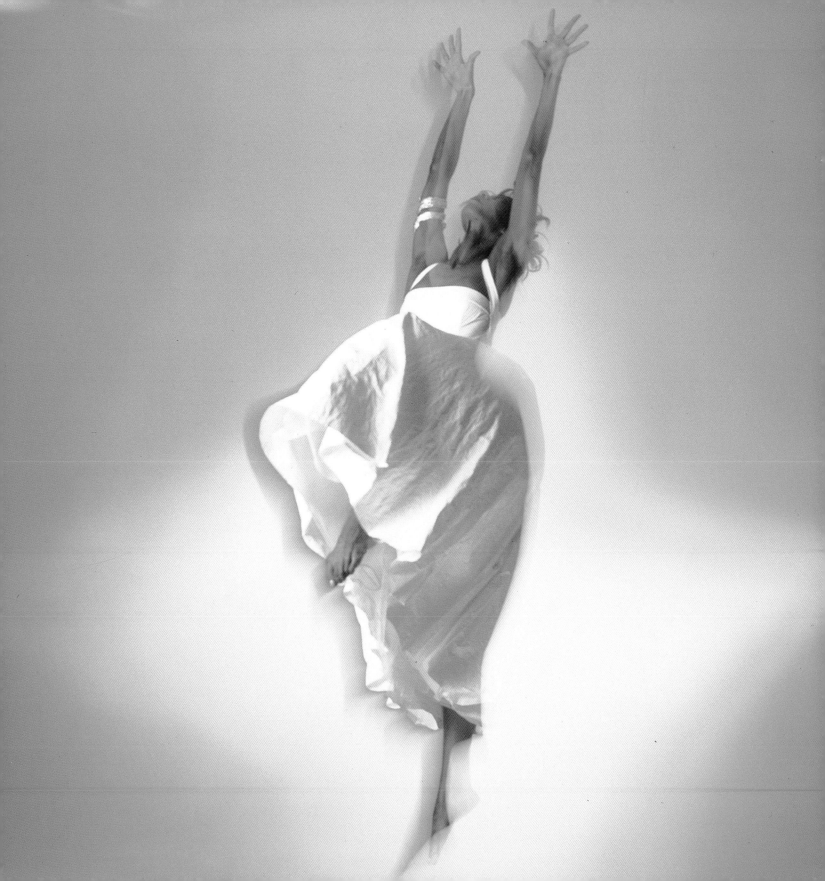

FOREWORD

BY PATRICIA MIGNON HINDS

My life has been a quest to learn and grow, in knowledge and in spirit. And there's always room to develop, learn more, and be better. For most of my life, I didn't comprehend the full meaning of *taking care of myself*. I had always automatically gravitated toward healthful activities and practices, such as sports and exercise, a more natural approach to makeup, and a do-it-at-home-between-touchups less-stress hairdo. But it all caught up to me when my life became so frenzied I stopped playing tennis, and didn't spend quite as much time maintaining my natural bronze. Then I began to value what it takes for everything to run in sync, to work in balance and in harmony. It made me appreciate my mother on a deeper level.

Seemingly effortlessly, my mother always stayed in shape, monitored her eating habits, kept every hair impeccably in place, maintained flawless skin and makeup, and kept an upbeat attitude. I am now more astounded than ever—wondering how she kept it all together. Growing up, I didn't fully appreciate what efforts it took for my mother to look so good, or what it took for her to take care of herself—as well as my sister Gail and me. Now I recognize, it's not that easy! My mother Gloria is my inspirational touchstone—and I want my life to reflect her loving attention, strength, and positive outlook. I know I should think green salad instead of glazed doughnut when those hips start feeling or looking out of control, make sure those elbows have some lotion on them, and keep my mind and spirit in the right direction. It's about keeping

the right mindset and planning to live under an overriding philosophy. So even when I go astray, I will get back on track before too long. It all boils down to some basics—be good to yourself and others, eat right and exercise, and plan for some pampering.

Pampering is about feeling good, taking care, and loving. We all deserve our share, and we shouldn't deprive or neglect ourselves. We must make time to allow ourselves to relax, enjoy, and enhance our lives. Through some simple acts and attention, we can add a spring to our steps, a spark to our souls, find a renewed sense of peaceful serenity. It's amazing what a little fragrance from a jasmine candle will do while soaking in a warm, relaxing bath, or how much more energy we have and fit we feel after just a half-hour of swimming, or how peaceful yet strong we feel after quiet moments of prayer. The value of taking care and honoring ourselves is priceless.

I embraced this project with the passion and excitement that I'd want to feel for anything I have lived and breathed during its creation—to make it the best—with meaning, substance, and beauty. This beauty isn't about makeup, but about radiating on the outside a reflection of what's inside. It's about inner as well as outer beauty. *The Essence Total Makeover* is developed with that in mind—putting together all the pieces that it takes to be our best. As this book emerged from its cocoon, it's come to embrace, reflect, and celebrate all we are as unique originals. It's about optimal health, happiness, and wholeness—all we can be to take ourselves to a higher level. It evolved to be both a learning experience and to reflect my pursuit of how I try (with varying degrees of success) to live my life.

I have always been especially interested in keeping informed—from today's news and technology to ancient Egyptian history. And that's not a stretch when I realize how it all comes together—learning that many generations ago, our African ancestors tapped nature's resources for some of the same healing and beautifying sources that now have emerged as "breakthroughs." Like Egyptian kohl being used as eye shadow or liner. Or clay, as well as plants like aloe vera, being utilized by various African peoples—like the Yoruba and Ashanti—for healing and aesthetic aids. Or the Bororo people of West Africa and people of Kau in the Sudan, two groups of many who use natural colors found in ocher, ground shells, and ash. Or water being revered for its therapeutic, cleansing, and spiritual benefits among many cultures around the world. Some of their wisdom has been tapped to make this book both current and timeless.

Let's look at all the opportunities and possibilities there are for us. When the hair, skin, body, or spirit seems to be breaking down—and we all know what that means—let's think makeover time. When we conceive makeover, let's imagine rebirth or rejuvenation in those areas where we can use a little cleansing, fresh approaches, a new breath of life. Let's remember what we can do to become empowered and enlightened. Let's look at some of the steps we can take on our journeys to looking, feeling, and being our greatest and most powerful.

INTRODUCTION

BY SUSAN L. TAYLOR, EDITOR-IN-CHIEF, *ESSENCE* MAGAZINE

We sisters are the mothers of invention, not just because we cradled civilization—giving birth to language, culture, and community—but because we are masters at using whatever resources are available to us to fashion whatever we need. There was a time when the beauty products we have now were nowhere to be had, and the only lab creating cosmetics for women of color was the one we set up in our own kitchens. We mixed and stirred and blended Avon and Chanel with cocoa powder or ground cinnamon and Crisco. Thank God for all the products that are now right at our fingertips in the shades and textures that marry well with the rainbow of our beauty.

Today we have choices. Today we have a wider range of options and greater freedom than at any time in our history to improvise and define for ourselves who we are and *how we be.* We can wear our hair relaxed or natural or be naturally relaxed. We can go braided or bald or even blond. We can slim down, *volupt,* augment, or redistribute our real and imagined assets and liabilities. We can make up or be made over. We can choose our look and lifestyle or simply change our mind or attitude. We can change our life. We can reinvent ourselves, inside and out, anytime we choose. We can be fluid like music, moving harmoniously, creatively through the changes life challenges us with. And that's the real beauty of who we are.

From its inception, *Essence* has been dedicated to expanding the choices available to us in every aspect of our lives. The magazine was in fact created to provide Black women with options—alternatives to a universe of lifestyle and fashion magazines in which we could find no reflection of ourselves, no affirmation of our own beauty. That beauty is innate, essential; it radiates from within, across the full spectrum of our skin tones, hair textures, and body shapes and sizes. And that fundamental premise has been the starting point from which *Essence* has explored new products and techniques, classic style, and the latest trends in hair and makeup.

Over the years, *Essence* makeovers have been one of the most popular features in the magazine. (The very first makeover we ran was in fact a freelance project I did as a young cosmetologist and owner of a fledgling cosmetics company. It won me the job of beauty editor in 1971.) Of course it's been impossible to fill even a fraction of the thousands of requests we get each year from sisters who want beauty and whole-life makeovers. And so we offer you this guidebook. In the pages that follow we have put into your hands the knowledge and resources that we editors tap into each month to create those articles in the magazine that help us sisters to live fully and freely, healthfully and beautifully, head to toe, from the inside out. We want you to be able to create for yourself what we do on the pages of *Essence.* It's all here in more than a hundred beautiful photographs and a wealth of information gathered from celebrated beauties and beauty experts, delivered in articles and anecdotes; tips, techniques, and advice on beauty, health, and our spiritual and emotional well-being.

More than anything, this is a book about possibilities—about our unlimited potential for creativity and happiness once we assume the courage to be our true and best selves. What a blessing it is to be able to envision how and what we want to be in the world, then roll up our sleeves and do the work of bringing that vision into being. Anytime we choose, we can renew ourselves, we can begin again, we can change. But we first have to be honest with ourselves

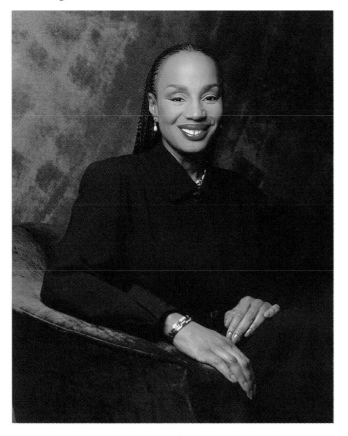

in assessing our strengths and weaknesses and in facing our fears. This may mean making peace with our hair, our color, our body—our unique beauty. It may mean scraping the scales from our eyes, left there by layer upon layer of popular images that narrowly define beauty and limit our vision of our own. Or recognizing the lies we were told as children about our looks, our size, our behavior, and, ultimately, our worth. It almost always means spending time in solitude and silence, getting in touch with that still, small voice within us that is God guiding us. When we are willing to look, and listen, we discover the truth that, in all the universe, this miracle of flesh and blood and breath and circumstances we see before us in the mirror is unique. Each of us is a divine original. Ultimately, we must discover that beauty is our birthright, it's the presence of God in us, that it is nowhere lacking and in fact infinite. It is our vision that is finite and weak. But it's never too late to open your eyes, to try to see yourself more clearly and develop an intense love and appreciation for the being you are.

This is a book about loving and honoring yourself just as you are. It's about recognizing that your beauty resides not in the art or techniques of makeup and styling but in your understanding of your wholeness and your vision of yourself as a creative being with art and techniques at your disposal, a world of resources, unlimited options, and the greatest gift that God has given you, your freedom to choose.

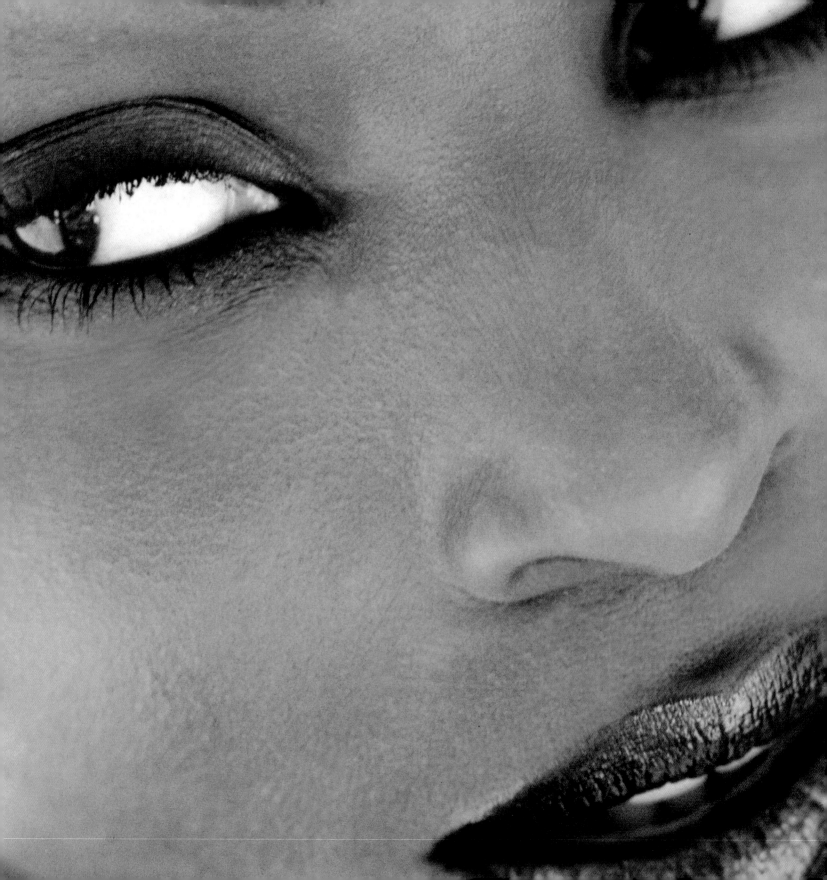

1

LOVING OUR SKIN

OUR SKIN IS A GIFT FROM MOTHER NATURE. It comes in a sumptuous spectrum of colors. From butterscotch to bronze to blackberry, people of color all over the world are naturally dipped in pretty and distinctive hues. What is so special about the rich colors of our skin? Our skin has been blessed from birth with an extra protective barrier against the lines, wrinkles, and other ravages of chronic sun abuse.

Melanin, the dark pigment in skin cells, gives our skin that extra protection, special tone, and helps us to stay younger-looking longer. While our skin is kissed with healthy properties, it is also prone to certain kinds of scarring, irritations, and other conditions. But there's nothing to worry about—it just means that caring for our complexion requires gentle and loving care.

GREAT SKIN

We're all on a quest for a smooth, radiant complexion. And we can have it by paying close attention to our skin's basic needs, adopting a simple, specific skin-care regimen and consulting experts when necessary.

First, you'll need to determine your skin type. But contrary to what a lot of beauty experts have espoused in the past, dividing skin into types—oily, dry, or combination—is only the first step. The truth is that your skin changes, sometimes on a daily basis depending on the climate, the season, the altitude, the foods you're eating, your health, and the stress in your life. On the right is a quiz to help you determine your general skin type. Also, note that any skin type can be sensitive.

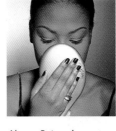

Above: Determine your skin type. *Below:* Our beauty is found in a range of sumptuous brown tones. *Opposite:* Exquisite bronze beauty.

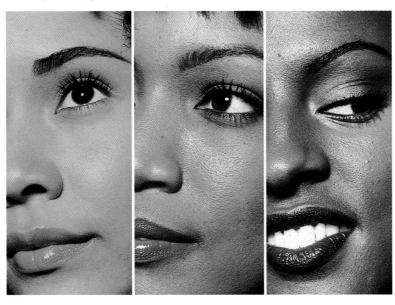

SELF-ASSESSMENT

- Do you cleanse your skin in the morning and by noon it s shiny all over?
- Do you have persistent adult acne or suffer from frequent breakouts such as random blackheads or whiteheads?
- Are your pores large and visible all over your face?
- Is your skin just as oily in the winter as it is during the rest of the year?

If you answered yes to most of these questions, your skin is most likely oily.

- Is your skin dry all over?
- When you look in the mirror, do you see fine tiny lines?
- Does your skin constantly flake during the winter months?
- Does washing your face with soap cause excessive dryness?
- Are your pores barely noticeable?

If you answered yes to most of these questions, your skin is probably dry.

- Does your skin appear shiny in the T-zone area forehead, nose, and chin but slightly dry on cheeks?
- Do you have large pores around the nose area but normal-size ones on the rest of your face?
- Is your skin drier in the winter and more oily in the summer?

If you answered yes to the majority of these questions, you have combination skin.

- When you wash your oily, dry, or combination skin with facial soap, does it cause irritation?
- Does your skin break out in a rash when using certain cosmetic products and fragrances?
- Is your skin prone to blotchy or reddish breakouts?

If you experience these concerns, you have sensitive skin.

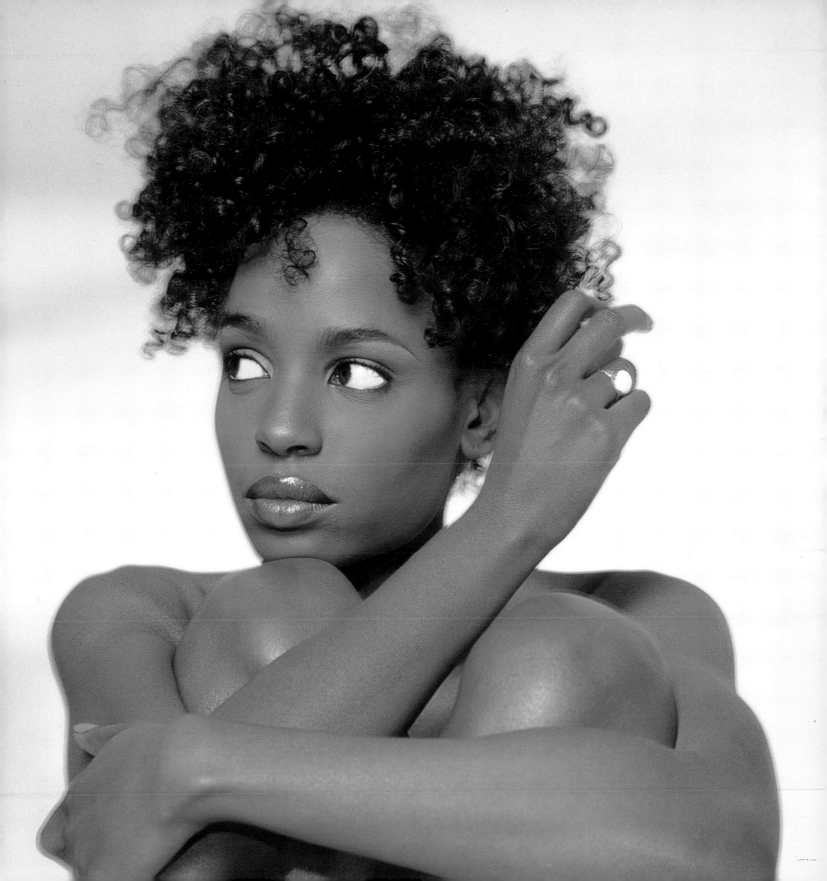

CARING FOR YOUR COMPLEXION

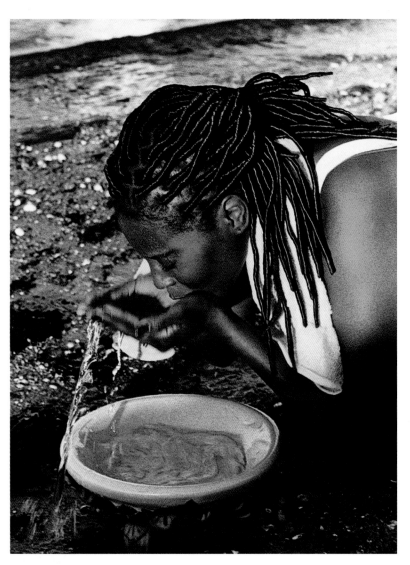

Basic skin care means cleansing (at least twice a day, morning and night), moisturizing (just as often), and sometimes using a toner or astringent—especially if your skin is oily, but not necessarily if it's on the dry side. In addition, you should protect your skin from sun damage and skin cancer with daily use of sunscreen.

Cleanse with Kindness

When you wash your face, cleanse your skin with an upward, circular motion, taking care not to pull or tug at the finer, more delicate skin around the eye area and throat. Some beauty experts suggest using a coarse washcloth—one that's only for washing your face —to provide a gentle exfoliating treatment that won't damage your skin. Exfoliation, by the way, simply means the removal of the dead cells that naturally build up on everyone's skin. Although invisible, these cells can make your skin look dull, dry, and older than it should if they do not shed properly. Remember, when shopping for beauty products, be sure to purchase products specifically formulated for your skin type.

• OILY complexions—can use softly-milled complexion bars or cleansing gels. Keep in mind that harsher isn't better: A too-harsh cleanser dries out the top layer of skin, causing irritation.

• DRY skin—opt for a facial cleanser formulated for dry skin or a creamy cleanser that rinses off with water during winter months. (Tissue-off cleansers generally leave a stubborn residue.)

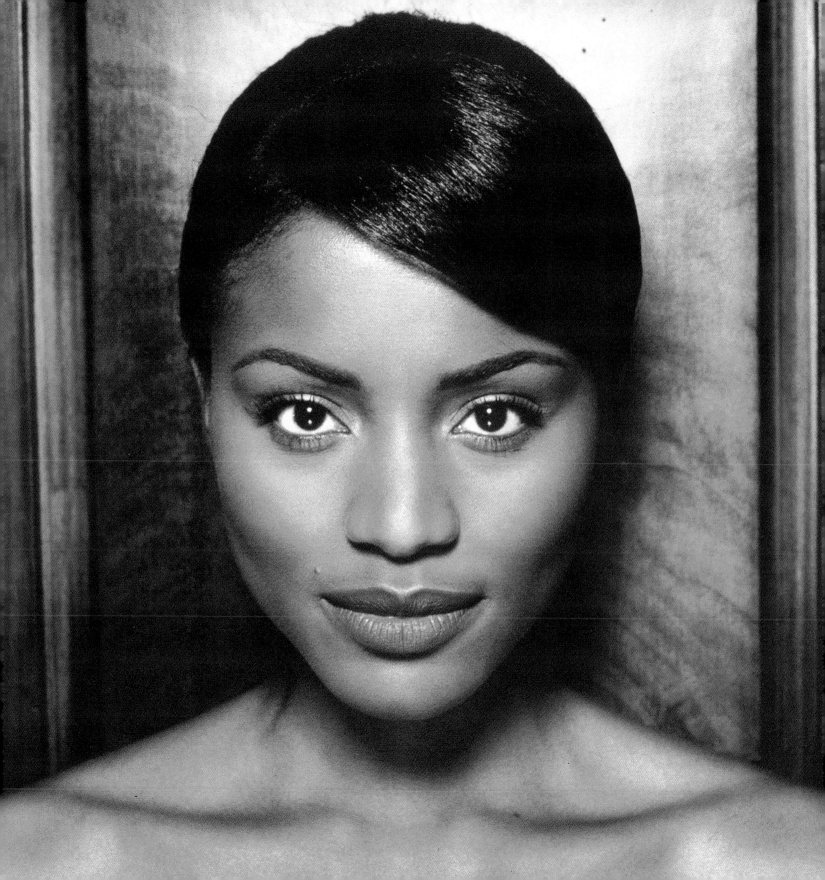

Alternate between creamy cleansers and cleansing gels during warmweather months. If your skin is especially dry and you're a non-makeup wearer, simply wash your face with water.

• SENSITIVE complexions—steer clear of facial scrubs and harsh cleansers. Limit steaming sessions (either at home, in saunas, or at health clubs) to two minutes, no longer.

Toners and Astringents

After cleansing, some women like to use a toner, freshener, or astringent to remove the last vestiges of makeup soot and soapy residue from the skin. Toners and fresheners are mild and contain no alcohol. Astringents containing alcohol can dry the surface of your skin and block impurities beneath the surface. Overdrying the skin (which in some instances can actually overstimulate oil production) is one of the biggest problems women with oily skin face. Whichever you prefer—toner or astringent—use it with an all-natural cotton ball or pad.

Moisturizers

Humectants in moisturizers help the skin stay supple by retaining its moisture as well as attracting water from the atmosphere. Dermatologists say that all types of skin benefit from moisturizers, even oily complexions, given that oil and water are two distinct elements. So how should you choose a moisturizer? Start with the most basic—unscented and free of lanolin and mineral oil. If your skin tends to

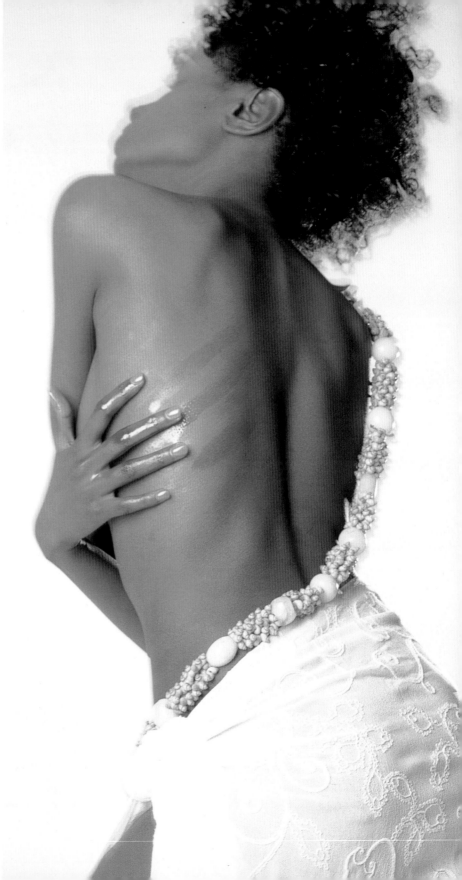

break out, try any of the oil-free brands or ask your skin therapist about a moisturizer made especially for oily skin, one that minimizes the appearance of large pores and leaves a matte finish. If your skin is dry, make sure your moisturizer is creamy. Use heavy moisturizers with caution though, because they sometimes contain acne-causing ingredients such as lanolin, petroleum jelly, and mineral oil. If you're prone to fine lines under the eyes—not uncommon as we age—be sure to dab a little moisturizer on the outer corners of the eyes.

Alpha Hydroxy Acids (AHAs)

Some scientific evidence suggests that alpha hydroxy acids, which come from fruit and milk sugars, are beneficial to our skin. What exactly do they do? Cosmetics with AHAs perform a less intense version of chemical peeling, a procedure dermatologists and plastic surgeons perform in the office. AHAs reportedly help improve the look of the skin by sloughing off discolorations, rough skin, and fine lines—all signs of aging skin. The chemicals cause the skin to shed its outer layers, revealing a fresher-looking layer of skin.

AHAs (often in the form of glycolic and lactic acids) can now be found in an increasing array of skin-care products, including cleansers, toners, moisturizers, serums, peels, and body lotions. But users should take extra care with these products. Since you're actually putting acids on the skin, it follows that use

of these products would raise questions of consumer safety. The Food and Drug Administration (FDA) warns that the use of AHA products can cause a greater sensitivity to the sun, raising the risk of photoaging and skin cancer, so use them with sunscreen. Studies have also found that some women have reported adverse reactions to AHA products, including mild irritations, stinging, blistering, and burning. If you have even the mildest reaction, discontinue use immediately.

When you want to try a new product containing these acids, test it by rubbing a dab in the crook of your elbow and leaving it undisturbed for forty-eight hours. Then test it again. If you don't notice a reaction, proceed with facial application. If you do experience

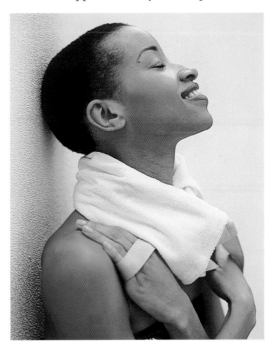

I HAVE VERY DRY SKIN SO IT NEEDS TO BE CONSTANTLY EXFOLIATED TO REMOVE DEAD SKIN CELLS. ONCE A WEEK I USE AN ALPHA HYDROXY ACID MOISTURIZING PEEL.

some irritation, dermatologists suggest waiting up to twenty minutes after cleansing before applying an AHA.

Pores

Our pores produce and disperse sweat and the oils that protect skin from the environment, much the same way tears protect the delicate tissue of the eye area. Without pores, oils from the sebaceous glands would be trapped underneath the skin. No amount of cleaning or treatment can shrink pores smaller than your genetically programmed size, but you can keep them clean. Pore strips claim to pick up dead skin cells that haven't shed properly and have formed a "plug" that's imbedded in pores. Don't pin your hopes on these strips;

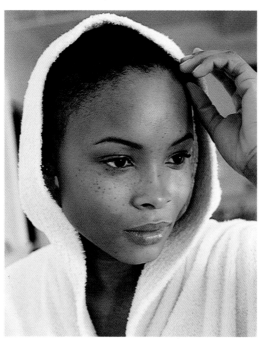

Right: The long-lasting glow from a relaxing visit to the spa.
Opposite: Erykah Badu.

many experts question their effectiveness.

A time-honored method for pore perfection is steaming. For years, this has been touted as a "pore opener," but that's not exactly true. What steaming actually does is soften the skin through superhydration. Softer skin may more easily release impurities and look slightly plumper, which helps to create a healthy glow.

Lip Care

Because lips are one of the most exposed areas of the body, they often show signs of overexposure, such as dryness, chapping, and cracking. They are sensitive because they consist primarily of a thin mucous membrane that has to work hard to fight off irritants like pollution and ultraviolet rays from the sun. Lips can benefit from moisturizers, sunscreens, and certain alpha hydroxy treatments—exfoliating creams designed specifically for lips—that remove dry skin overnight and gently refine.

Facials

Skin-care authorities vary in their position on facials. Some experts will tell you they are not necessary for the maintenance of good skin. Others will say that like exercising, facials can help stimulate blood circulation and the flow of oxygen to purge skin of the toxins imbedded in pores. Some women depend on them anywhere from bimonthly to several times a year, and either go to an aesthetician for one or do it themselves at

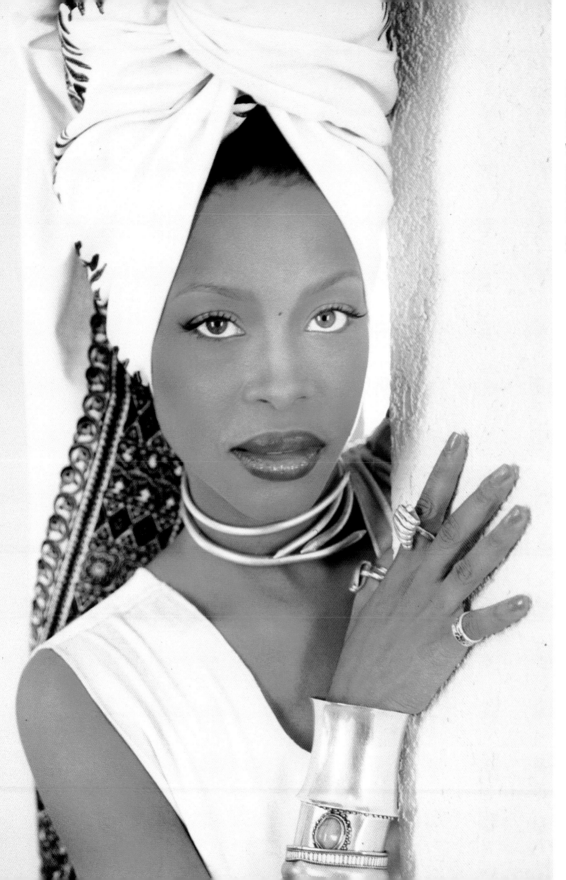

ERYKAH BADU
I MOISTURIZE
MY FACE WITH
VITAMIN E
EVERY NIGHT.
I FIND IT
GIVES MY SKIN
A SMOOTH
TEXTURE.

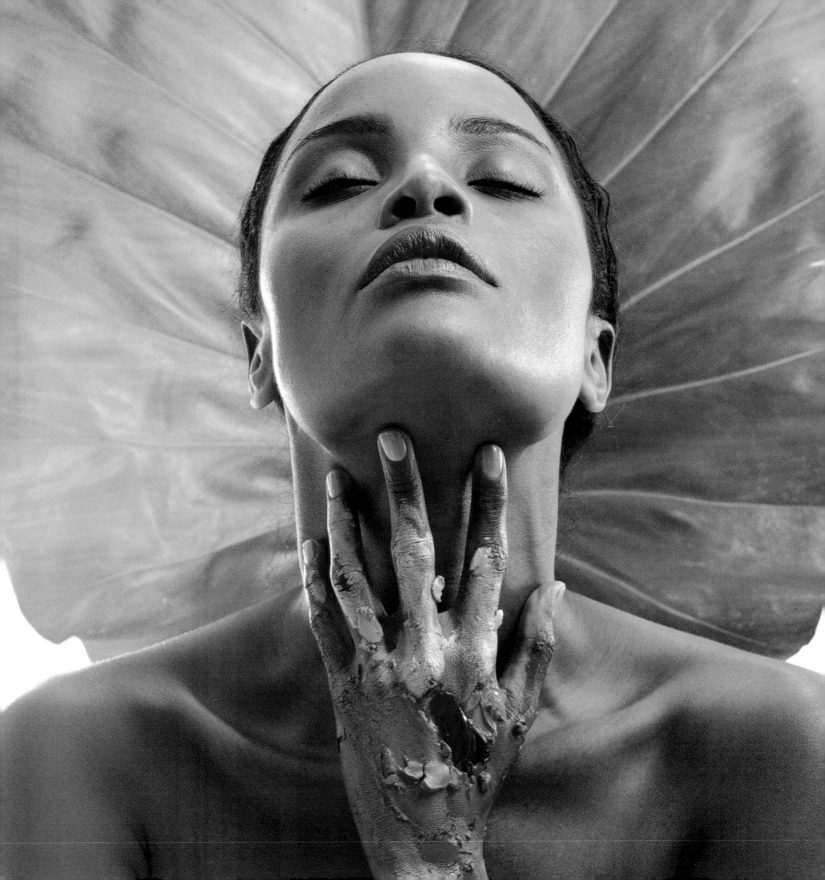

home. The only thing all experts seem to agree on is that facials are soothing and wonderfully relaxing. Let your skin be your guide, however, and keep in mind that less stress on facial skin is always better.

One of the benefits of a professional facial is that it's accompanied by a gentle face, neck, and often shoulder massage.

Depending on your skin type as well as your skin's needs, your skin-care therapist may prescribe any of the following:

• GLYCOLIC ACID FACIAL—a strong exfoliant session and hydrating facial for replenishing dehydrated skin

• DEEP-CLEANSING FACIAL—includes expert facial manipulation by the therapist and is good for cleaning out blackheads

• LYMPHATIC DRAINAGE FACIAL—a series of movements that begin over the eyebrow and are meant to activate your body's own toxin-fighting systems

• OXYGEN FACIAL—this latest addition to the facial family sends a jet of oxygen to help the skin regain its glow

Some professionals believe many of these facials are simply gimmicks. Again, you be the judge and remember that all you really need to take care of your skin is a good, basic cleansing ritual that works for you. Everything else is mere topping on the toast.

DES'REE
I SPEND A LOT OF TIME TRAVELING SO I DON'T LEAVE HOME WITHOUT COCOA BUTTER. I SLATHER IT ON MY FACE, BODY, AND HAIR.

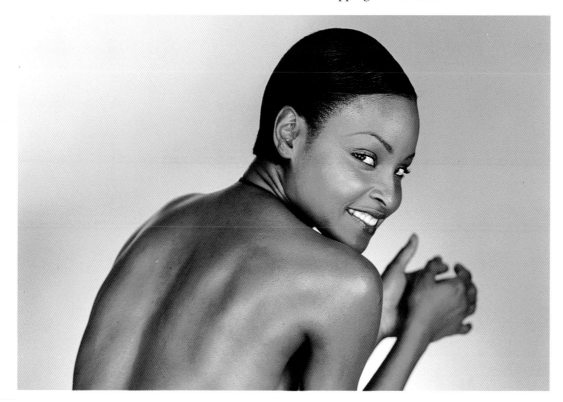

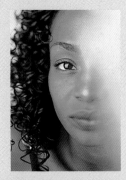

Above: Understanding your skin type is an important step of a skin-care regimen. *Opposite:* Model Patrice Jordan uncovers the beauty of her skin.

NATURAL SKIN-CARE MASKS

While there are many commercial masks available over-the-counter, you can concoct your own skin-revitalizing or healing recipes using the most basic food items. You're the head chef in this beauty kitchen.

DRY SKIN

AVOCADO MASK Create a nourishing mask from the mashed-up pulp of an avocado, which is full of proteins and amino acids. Apply it all over your face and throat, wait a few minutes, then rinse.

PROTEIN MASK Egg whites also nourish dry and sensitive skin. Apply beaten egg whites and let dry; leave on for fifteen minutes, then rinse.

OILY AND COMBINATION SKIN

BANANA MASK Go fruity. Mash one whole banana in a small bowl. Add one tablespoon of honey and a few drops of orange or lemon juice. Mix to form a paste. Leave on for fifteen minutes, then rinse with warm water. Beauty benefits: Banana calms the skin, and orange juice with its fruit acid benefits can remove the superficial layer of flaky, dry skin. You can also try peaches, strawberries, or white grapes.

ACNE MASKS Pastes made with herbs and spices can reduce inflammation, bacteria, and excess oil. Blend equal amounts of fresh mint and coriander in a food processor. Or grind half a teaspoon of dried yellow lentils and mix with a teaspoon of water to create a paste. Holistic experts suggest adding powdered zinc (which can be purchased at any health food store) to any of the above recipes; it will increase the anti-inflammatory benefits and hold the mixture together better.

AT-HOME STEAM TECHNIQUE

1 gallon water
2 tablespoons salt
¾ cup peppermint leaves
1 bowl
1 towel
facial mask (optional)
toner
sage (optional)
witch hazel (optional)

Boil water, adding two tablespoons of salt per gallon. Pour the boiling water over the peppermint leaves in an unheated, temperature-safe bowl (to avoid burning yourself during steaming). Place your face twelve inches above the water, and use a towel to cover your head like a tent to keep the steam in. Alternate two minutes of steaming over the bowl with a two-minute break.

Be careful not to stay too long over the steam. Repeat this cycle up to five times for a total of ten minutes over the steam. Rinse your face in room-temperature water. This is a good time to use a mud or peel-off facial mask to get the maximum benefit while your pores are open.

Rinse your face again. Follow with a toner or astringent. You can even make your own natural toner with one cup of dried garden sage leaves and two cups of witch hazel.

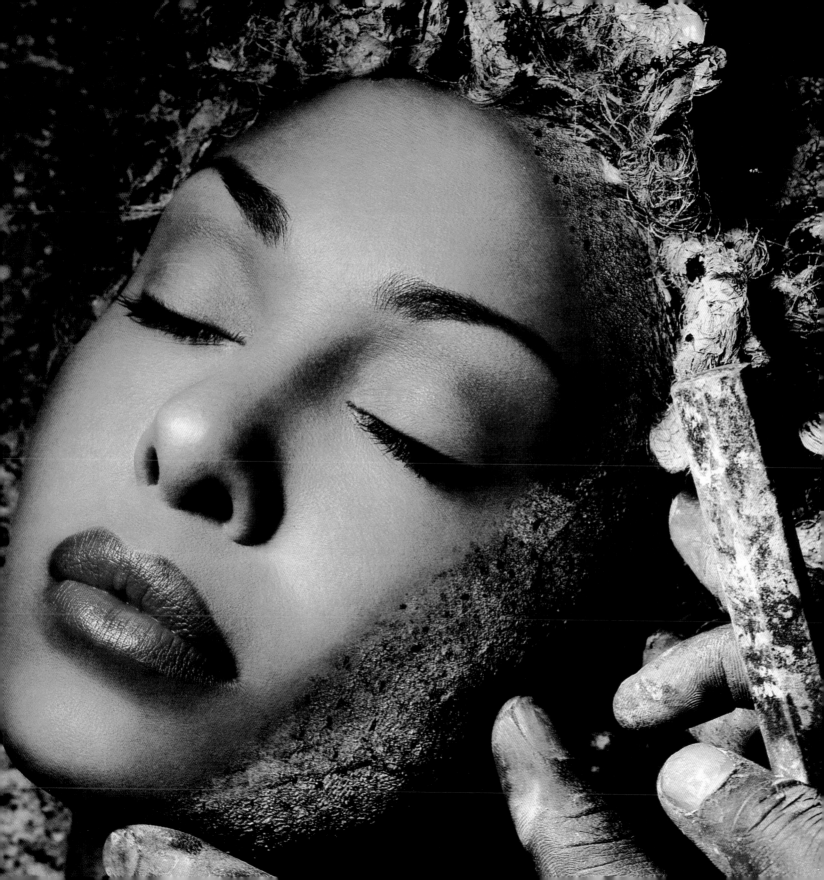

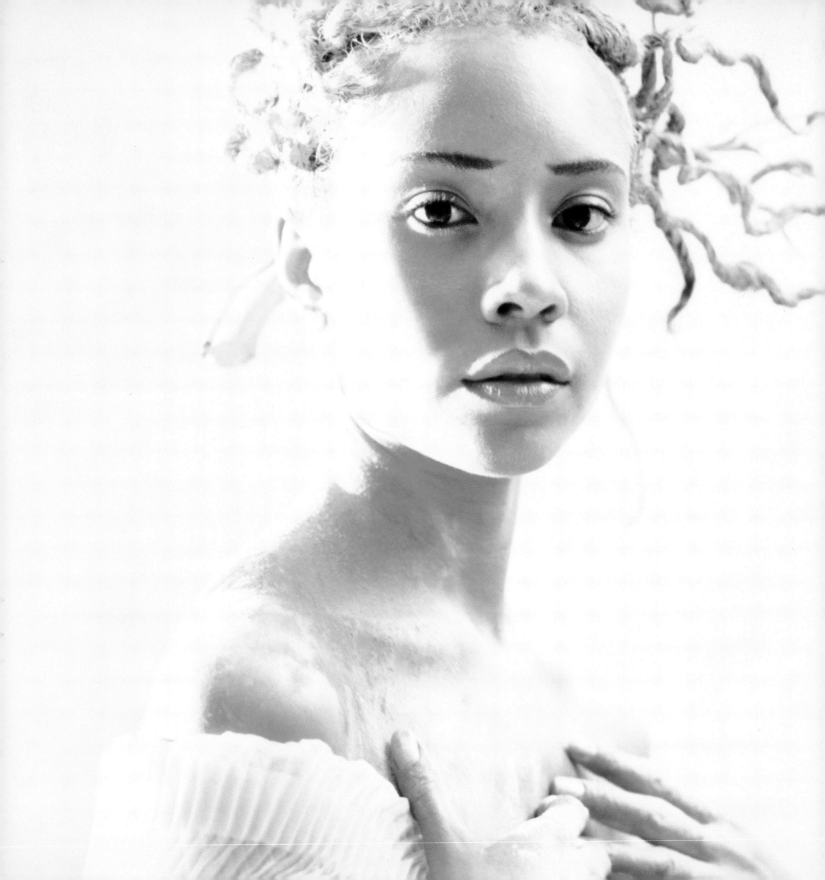

SKIN 911

Skin, the body's largest organ, has its own particular sensitivities. How many times have you awakened with puffy eyes, an unwelcome zit, or found your skin "well done" from sitting in the sun all day? No doubt there are a myriad of influences (pollution, chemicals in foods, the ozone layer) that cause our skin problems. Here are a few real-deal facts and solutions for coping with your skin when it's facing too much stress.

Acne

This problem develops when the sebaceous glands begin to work overtime, as they do in adolescence, making the skin more oily. When the pores are blocked, dead cells, bacteria, and sebum accumulate, forming a plug.

TO WARD OFF BREAKOUTS Don't over-cleanse your face or use harsh cleansers. Vigorous washing and scrubbing will actually irritate the skin and make acne worse. Stick to gentle choices such as an oil-free acne wash or beauty soap bar. Follow with an oil-free and lanolin-free moisturizer. Stress and poor diet might trigger the acne if you are already prone. Taking care of yourself, anyway, is never bad advice: Eat a well-balanced, healthy diet; get enough sleep; and drink lots of water. To reduce everyday stress, begin regular cardiovascular exercise to keep circulation revved up, and start yoga or meditation to promote relaxation. Try drinking herbal teas such as burdock or dandelion, known for their detoxifying and liver-cleansing properties. Increasing your intake of vitamin A acts to normalize skin and helps keep oil production in check. Zinc can reduce inflammation, redness, and swelling. Beta-carotene can boost the immune system and increase resistance to infection. For the prevention of preperiod flare-ups, try taking vitamin B_6 twice a day during the week prior to your period, and then during the week of your period. This helps to combat the stress, hormonal havoc, and the increased oil production that comes along for the ride.

WHAT TO DO IF YOU WAKE UP WITH BLACKHEADS OR WHITEHEADS After cleansing, apply a medicated gel or cream that contains salicylic acid or benzoyl peroxide. If you have dozens of breakouts or severe acne, it's best to get a thorough pore extraction by a dermatologist. Your dermatologist will also prescribe an appropriate skin-care regimen (bring all of your beauty products with you), topical prescription treatments, and, if necessary, oral antibiotics.

FOR SERIOUS CYSTIC ACNE The newest topical treatment is a salicylic or a beta hydroxy acid peel that's done in a doctor's office. If peels are scheduled on a regular basis, blockages are dissolved and oil production is kept in check. A consultation with a dermatologist will determine if you are indeed a candidate for a chemical peel. Also effective are cortisone injections, which shorten the life span of a cyst from two to three weeks to just a few days; in fact, swelling goes down substantially within a day.

WHAT TO AVOID IF YOU'RE ACNE-PRONE
Do not wear makeup with Red D and C dyes, especially blushes and lipsticks, and remove all makeup before going to bed. It's also important to wash your hands frequently and keep them off your face, and to change your pillowcase frequently (twice a week), so the residue from hair products doesn't end up on your face.

Canker Sores

Not to be confused with cold sores, which are highly contagious viral sores on the outside of your mouth, canker sores are small, painful sores that usually occur on the inside of the lip or cheek or under the tongue. Experts think they may be caused by bacteria, irritation of the area, stress, or allergies. *Action alert:* If you experience any other symptoms (fever, fatigue, weight loss) you should see a doctor—a more serious condition could be causing the sores.

Dark Circles

If lack of sleep isn't the culprit (you need between seven to nine hours a night), then dark circles under your eyes could be due to stress, improper diet, or they may be hereditary. Today's alpha hydroxy acids have had considerable success in lightening dark circles, but they should only be used under a derma-

tologist's supervision. You can also try using green tea bags. Boil them, put them in the refrigerator, and place cold bags over your eyes. This may reduce swelling and relieve your eyes.

Eczema

This is a chronic skin inflammation and is commonly contracted by those who are prone to allergies such as hay fever, seasonal allergies, and asthma. What does it look like? Dry and itchy skin, or scaly red patches of skin that show up anywhere on the face or body. Those with eczema should use only mild body cleansers labeled as moisturizing and nonirritating (exfoliants and scrubs are out), followed by super-rich moisturizers. A dermatologist might prescribe a topical steroid cream and perhaps an antihistamine to treat the reaction. For mild cases of eczema, ask your pharmacist to recommend an over-the-counter anti-inflammatory ointment or cream.

Facial Hair

Medical alert: Excess hairiness can be a sign of an underlying medical problem; clearing up the problem beforehand with help from a dermatologist or endocrinologist can make any hair-removal treatment much more successful.

WAXING removes hairs slightly below the surface and encourages a softer, nonstubby regrowth.

DEPILATORIES should never be used on eyebrows or other areas around the eyes where

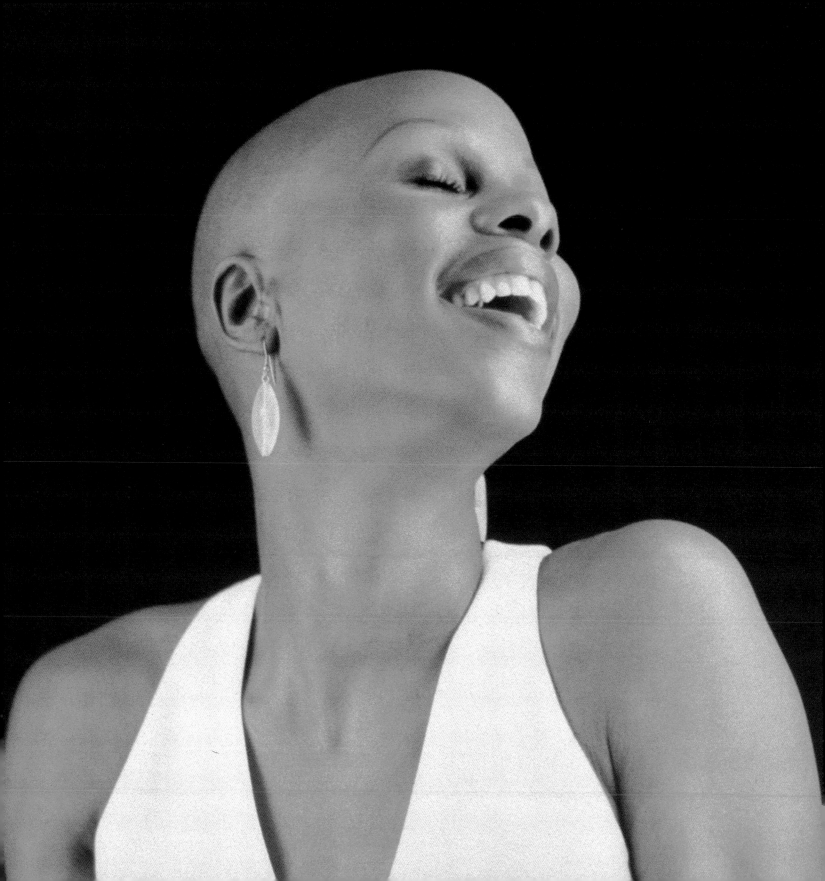

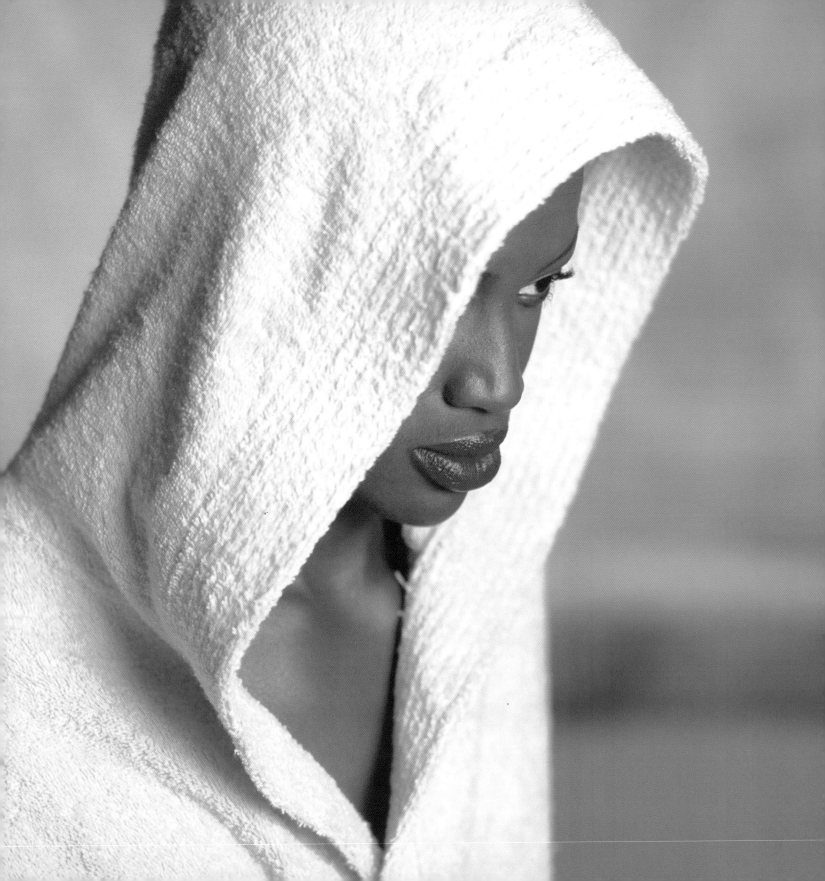

they can cause severe skin irritations. Think about it: The active ingredient most commonly used in depilatories is calcium thioglycolate, which is also used in hair relaxers. (Imagine that on your face!) When treating the face or bikini lines, use depilatories specifically labeled for those areas.

ELECTROLYSIS Because of the time-consuming nature and expense of the process, electrolysis is only recommended for hair removal on small areas. A thin needle is inserted into the hair follicle and a mild electric current passes through to weaken hair at its growth source. The hair is then removed with tweezers. If it sounds painful, that's because it can be. Done properly, electrolysis may leave the skin slightly red immediately after treatment, or with a very small amount of scabbing. Even the most skilled electrologist cannot guarantee that it will not scar darker complexions. Anyone who has a heart condition or is prone to skin conditions such as eczema or psoriasis should not have electrolysis without first checking with a physician.

LASER SURGERY Some dermatologists are now using lasers to remove hair. The technique selectively targets the pigment in the hair follicle and destroys it. Though the jury is still out, results are said to be similar to those for electrolysis—that is, it often takes several treatments, and the hair eventually grows back. The problem for Black women lies in the fact that the laser also picks up the pigment in the top layer of the skin, changing the skin color in the process of removing the hair.

SHAVING should not be considered an option for sisters with coarse, curly hair because of the risk of ingrown hairs. Women with problem-free skin, clear complexions, and faint facial hair are the best candidates for shaving.

Facial Warts

Anyone can be exposed to warts—they're viral growths that are very contagious and therefore can be transferred through skin contact such as kissing or shaking hands. There are two kinds of warts: flat, flesh-colored bumps and "cauliflower"–looking moles. Both can be treated with over-the-counter salicylic acid products. If they don't respond, a dermatologist can treat them with topical chemicals or remove them surgically. Sometimes they even go away on their own.

Flesh Moles

About one-third of all African-Americans have "flesh moles." These brown or black, sometimes raised, hereditary growths—about as large as a pencil point—are totally harmless unless they change color or appearance, which could be a sign of skin cancer. They often begin appearing on the cheeks and necks of women in their early thirties and are common in middle-aged or older people. If they bother you, a dermatologist can easily clip them or remove them with an electric needle.

Hyperpigmentation

Darker spots, which can be caused by every-thing from acne (made worse by picking and squeezing pimples), mosquito bites, burns, and sun damage can be worrisome. But not to worry: Hyperpigmentation can naturally fade over time without medicine, and there are things you can do in the meantime to speed up the process. Try over-the-counter fade or bleaching products containing approximately 2 percent hydroquinone, the most commonly used bleaching agent. The latest products now combine hydroquinone with glycolic acid. The most important step when treating hyperpig-mentation spots, however, is rigorous protec-tion from the sun. Simply put: You must wear a sunscreen even during winter months or the condition may worsen.

Keloids

Scars on Black skin can take longer to fade and can "overheal," resulting in thickened raised scars, called keloids, that have extended and spread beyond the size of the original wound. Keloids can develop from anything that breaks the skin: ear piercing, insect bites, paper cuts, acne, or even minor medical procedures like the removal of a mole. If you're prone to keloids (and not every Black person is), they're most common on the chest, back, and earlobes. Some can be treated depending on the age, size, and location of the keloid. There are now products on the market that have been proven

effective in shrinking even old raised scars. Ask your pharmacist to recommend one.

Mask of Pregnancy

This is a skin condition that occurs during pregnancy and causes a darkening on the fore-head and cheeks. Mask of pregnancy, also known as melasma, is caused by hormonal activity and usually disappears after giving birth. Pregnant women may also experience other skin changes related to hormonal changes: darkening of moles, the growth of skin tags on the neck, or the darkening of facial moles. It's important that you use a moisturizer, wear a sunblock during the day, and take prenatal vitamins.

Menopausal Skin

During menopause, which occurs around the age of fifty, facial skin gradually becomes thin-ner, drier, and more fragile. Some women will experience an increase in facial hair, darkening of freckles, and the appearance of age spots (most noticeable in sisters with lighter to medium complexions). What's recommended: moisturizers with sunscreen during the day and the application of tretinoin or alpha hydroxy acid moisturizers at night to improve skin texture.

Skin Allergies

An allergy is a hypersensitivity of the body to certain agents, or allergens, it perceives as harm-

Right: Preventive maintenance keeps your skin healthy.

ful. Most allergens are harmless, but sometimes people respond to them with mild to severe reactions, discomfort, and coldlike symptoms.

ALLERGIC CONTACT DERMATITIS results in skin eruptions, rashes, or irritations when an offending agent comes in contact with the skin. The sun, dyes, plants, clothing, metal compounds, and ingredients in certain cosmetics and medications can all cause sensitivity. Inflamed, red, itchy patches or blisters on the skin can be treated by the application of topical corticosteroid cream and prevented by avoiding the allergen.

HIVES appear on the skin as red, raised, swollen, and itchy welts almost immediately after exposure to the allergen. Drugs like penicillin; certain foods such as fish, nuts, eggs, and milk; or the exposure to other allergens like pollen, animal dander, and insects can bring on attacks. To relieve the problem: Determine the cause of the reaction and avoid the allergen. Also, antihistamines and corticosteroids—topical or oral—can help.

Skin Cancer

The brown pigment that colors our skin, melanin, helps to block out skin-damaging sun rays. Despite this help from Mother Nature, we are still at risk for developing melanoma, the deadliest form of skin cancer. Black people tend to develop this cancer on the palms of the hands, soles of the feet, under nails, or in the mouth, but skin cancer

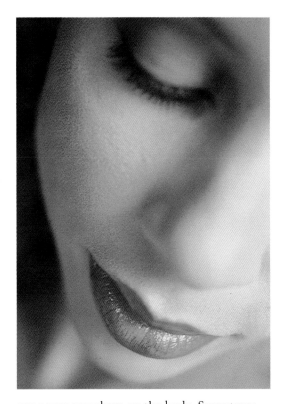

can occur anywhere on the body. Symptoms that are suspect and should be brought to the attention of your physician: a sore that doesn't heal, rapid change in the size or color of an existing mole, any new red spots that won't disappear, or any new discoloration. Other warning signs include: scaliness, oozing, bleeding, or the appearance of a bump or nodule; the spread of pigment from the border into surrounding skin; and a change in sensation including itchiness, tenderness, or pain. Atypical moles, which may run in families, can also serve as markers, identifying the person as being at higher risk for developing melanoma.

Have your skin examined by your general physician during your yearly checkup. Dermatologists also recommend that one helpful way to guard against skin cancer is to do periodic self-examinations. Get familiar with your skin and your own pattern of moles, freckles, and "beauty marks." Be alert to changes in the number, size, shape, and color of pigmented areas. If you notice any changes see your dermatologist. In addition, wear an SPF (sun protection factor) sunscreen of at least 15 when you're out in the sun. When used correctly, sunscreens can block ultraviolet rays and reduce the chances of serious burns.

Skin Tags

These tiny chunks of excess skin are generally harmless; they develop as a result of heredity, aging, pregnancy, obesity, or diabetes. The best treatment, if they bother you, is to have them removed by a dermatologist.

Vitiligo

A skin condition that results from loss of melanin, vitiligo is more noticeable on darker complexions than lighter ones, but occurs with equal frequency in individuals of all races. The root of the problem: Pigment is simply not produced in cells called melanocytes. The cause of vitiligo is unknown, but it generally appears around the eyes, lips, nose, tips of fingers, or on elbows and knees. Some people gradually lose pigment over their entire bod-

ies. What to do? Dermatologists can administer skin therapy over a prolonged treatment period to restore melanin production, but not all cases can be treated, especially those existing more than two years.

Wrinkles

In this case, an ounce of prevention is worth a pound of cure. While genetics play an important role in wrinkle formation, an unhealthy lifestyle will bring them on a lot sooner than you'd like. The culprits: smoking cigarettes, dehydration, drinking more than two glasses of alcoholic beverages a day, sleep deprivation, overexposure to the sun, and not using sufficient sunscreens and moisturizers.

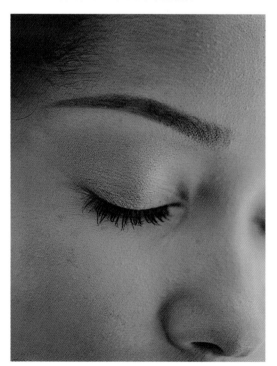

Below: Simplicity is the key to skin care and makeup. *Opposite:* Lasers can remove tattoos, moles, and other marks.

BREAK- THROUGHS OR BEAUTY MYTHS?

Collagen Treatments

The second deepest skin layer is the dermis, which is primarily composed of collagen, a valuable protein component of skin—that supplies it with suppleness, flexibility, and elasticity. There is no medical evidence, however, that beauty products containing collagen provide any benefits. On the other hand, collagen injections administered by a dermatologist or licensed plastic surgeon may improve the superficial appearance of wrinkles and deep furrows, with results lasting from three to six months. Anyone considering this procedure should act cautiously, because the injections can cause scarring on dark skin. Severe allergic reactions have been known to occur.

More on Laser Surgery

Laser treatments are being touted by dermatologists and plastic surgeons for everything from scar and unwanted hair removal to diminishing superficial wrinkles. The laser light flashes at one- to two-second intervals and vaporizes, cuts,

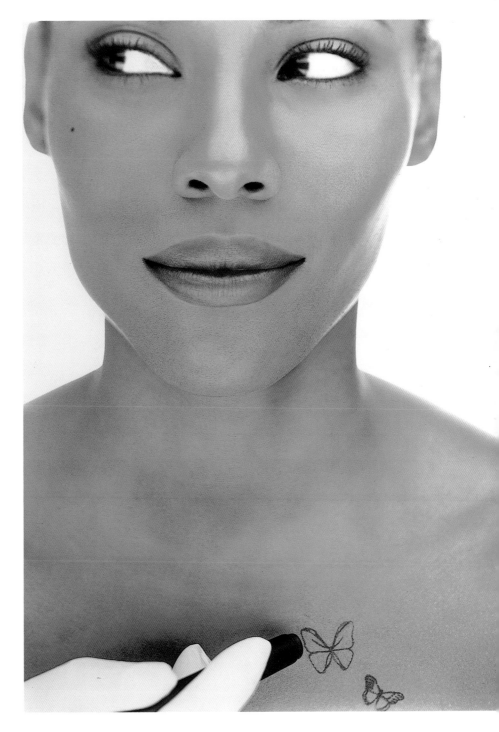

THE BEAUTY BAR

"Moisturizing products containing beta hydroxy acids (salicylic acids) are better for darker complexions than those containing alpha hydroxy acids (glycolic and lactic). The beta acids are made from wintergreen grass and are water soluble; this makes them gentler on the skin and less irritating while providing rapid exfoliation of the top layer of skin. What you're left with is a very healthy glow." —Irma Denson, Irma Denson Skin Care Salon and Day Spa, New York

"To deep cleanse your pores after cleansing and rinsing, take a warm washcloth and press it into your face for five minutes." —Dr. Beverly Johnson, dermatologist, Washington, D.C.

"The area around the eyes is said to be related to the kidney and gallbladder. If you have puffiness or dark circles you need to constantly drink water to flush out your kidneys. Dry complexions are further dehydrated by caffeine and smoking. It's important for coffee drinkers and smokers to drink a lot of water to flush the caffeine and nicotine out of their system." —Nona George Cohen, The Body Clinic, Los Angeles

"Breakouts are sometimes exercise-related. If you work out three to four times a week, you may notice the formation of fine little bumps on your forehead. What to do?
• Don't wear makeup when you're working out.
• Don't rub or touch your face with your hands. Make a habit of dabbing off sweat with a towel as often as you can during your workout.
• Wear a sweatband or scarf around your head to keep hair or facial products from running onto your face.
• Wash your face after a workout then head for the steam room and sweat out toxins from your pores at least once a week." —Dr. William D. Keith, Institute for Aesthetic and Cosmetic Dermatology, Los Angeles

"Don't overlook the wisdom and simplicity of our elders. Witch hazel, believe it or not, makes for a wonderful toner. It's very refreshing and not too drying on the skin." —Dr. Lynn McKinley-Grant, Washington Hospital Center in Washington, D.C., and American Academy of Dermatology

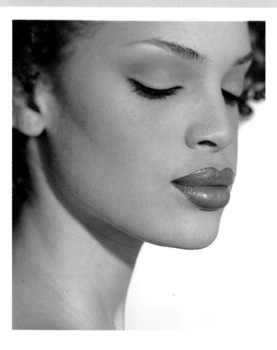

or seals the top layer of the skin, where imperfections are most visible. The question is does this technology work for us? How well a laser works depends on variables like the condition being treated, the laser used, and the skin type. Darker skins, for example, are at a higher risk of developing dark spots after surgery. And scars less than a year old are not good laser candidates because the body's own healing process takes a year. Treatments are costly and comparable results may be achieved with less expensive therapies. Warts, skin lesions, and tattoos are some of the newest targets to go under the laser. A dermatologist can determine if a specific concern of yours should be treated with a laser.

Left: Some experts recommend vitamin B$_6$ to curb pre-period flare-ups. *Opposite:* Darker skins are not immune to the ravages of the sun.

Chemical Peels

Despite the progress of chemical peels over the last decade, this surgical procedure, which involves removing the top layer of facial skin, can cause a local sensitivity and yield unwanted discolorations on certain complexions. Consult with a dermatologist first to see if you are a candidate for chemical peels. Make sure the doctor has had sufficient experience performing peels on dark skin. *Buyers beware:* Although facial therapists provide a version of superficial chemical peels with alpha hydroxy products, only a licensed dermatologist or plastic surgeon can perform deeper chemical peels.

Vitamin C Skin Care

The vitamin C we absorb naturally through foods is an antioxidant, and has been proven to protect the skin against ultraviolet light exposure and sun damage, but the jury is still out on whether vitamin C-laden skin products actually protect us. Using large amounts of vitamin C on the skin could prove useful in protecting it from the sun's harmful rays, which are the main culprits in skin aging and skin cancer. When selecting vitamin C skin-care products it's important to check the ingredient list. Vitamin C is ascorbic acid. For the highest concentration it must be listed as active or high on the list of ingredients. But remember, vitamin C is not a sunscreen and should be used in conjunction with a sunscreen product.

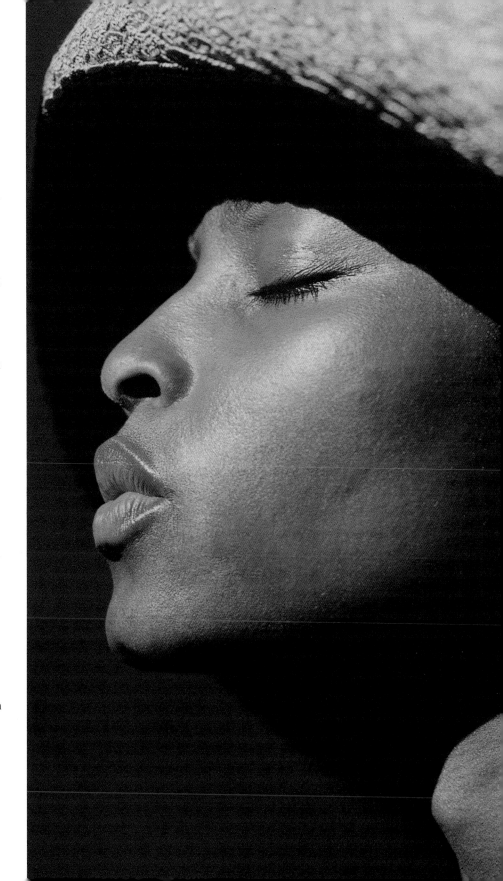

MAKEUP
BASIC TOOLS OF THE BEAUTY TRADE

Making up isn't hard to do if you have the right tools. What you'll need: sponge wedges that don't crumble and brushes that won't wilt before the job is done. Sable, pony, or natural

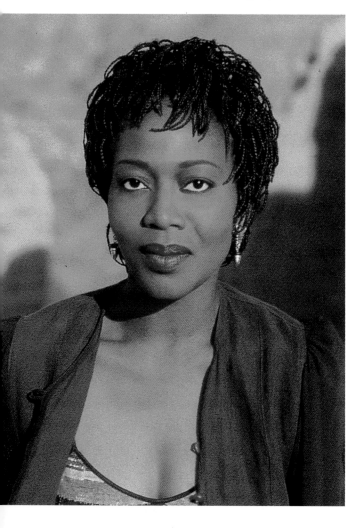

ALFRE WOODARD

MY EYES ARE BIG AND SOMETIMES PUFFY. TO CREATE MORE DEPTH I USE BROWN EYE SHADOW IN THE CREASE. TO CALM DOWN THE PUFFINESS WHEN I'M WORKING I TAKE WET TEA BAGS AND PLACE THEM ON MY LIDS FOR FIVE MINUTES BEFORE MAKEUP APPLICATION.

brushes will provide the longest use and precision strokes. Upkeep cues: Wash your brushes once a month in warm, soapy water, then let them dry naturally. While we don't suggest you purchase every single tool, we wanted you to have a look at the many options.

• SPONGES Blend concealer and foundation with absorbent sponge wedges for a more refined finish.

• POWDER BRUSH This is a hands-down favorite over the gargantuan powder puff preferred by movie makeup artists because it leaves behind the lightest "dusting," instead of a thick layer. The powder brush is the best for applying loose translucent powder over foundation or on bare skin.

• BLUSH BRUSH Invest in a sable or pony-haired brush for a more muted, professional application of blush.

• ROUND EYE SHADOW BRUSH A softly rounded brush like this one is perfect for highlighting along the brow bone to achieve a more prominent arch of the brow.

• EYEBROW BRUSH A stiff-bristled, slanted brush is used with brow powder to fill in sparse areas of the brow.

• LIP BRUSH Although you'll apply lipstick most of the time straight out of the tube, a lip brush will come in handy when you're spreading a lighter shade over a darker one, or simply desiring the most precise application possible.

Left: Alfre Woodard, actress. *Opposite:* A full arsenal of brushes adds a professional touch.

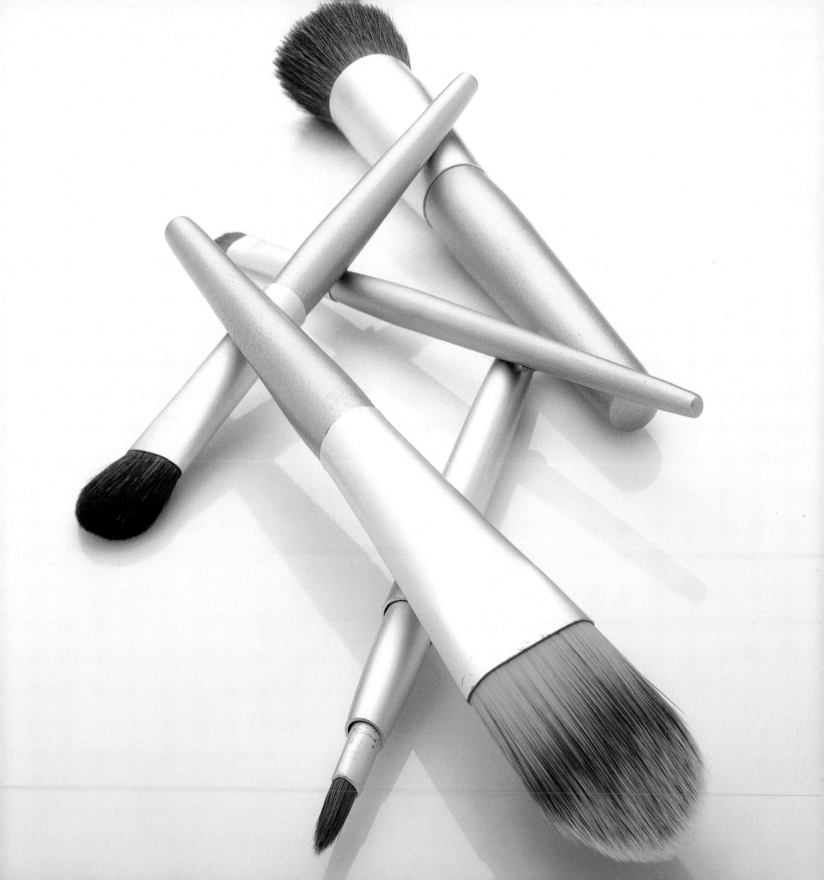

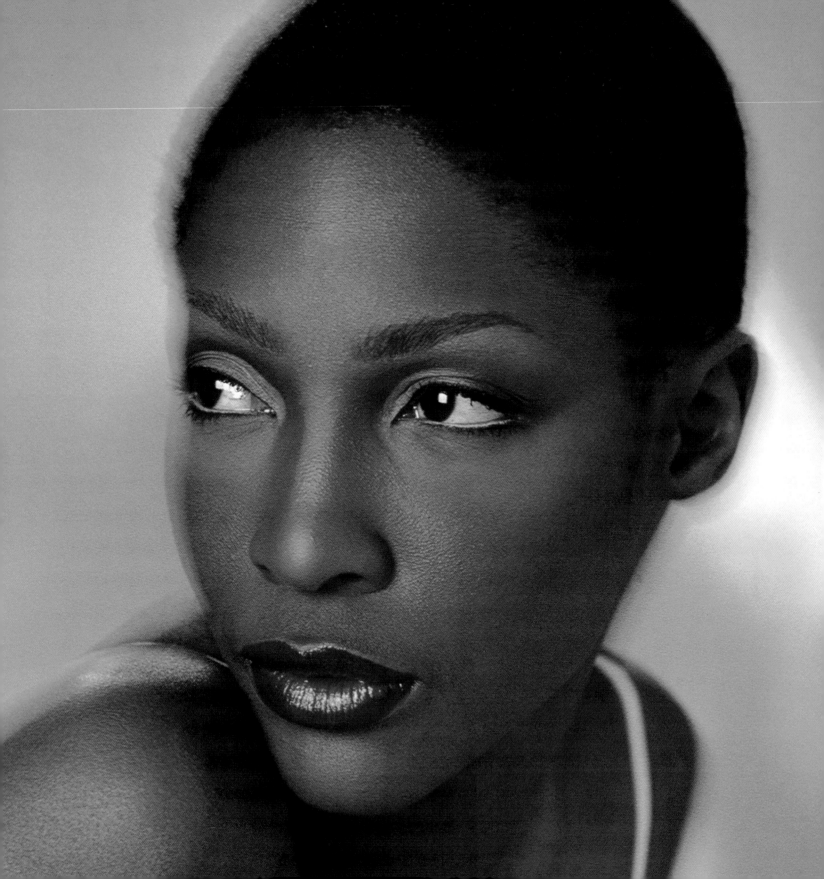

COVER YOUR BASES

CONCEALER Makeup artists say it all starts with concealer, which was created to cover blemishes, dark areas, undereye circles, and blotchy or ruddy spots. Today, concealer comes in wand formulas, pots, sticks, and even liquid. Concealers should generally be one shade lighter than your skin tone in order to camouflage those dark areas you want to even out. Your under eye area is naturally thinner and less resilient and thus more prone to cakiness than any other part of your face. To get a smoother look give it a pat with a makeup sponge.

FOUNDATION The right foundation depends on the depth and tone of your skin tone. Shade cues: Light-skinned women should look for a soft golden foundation. Medium-toned skin can wear shades with a red-yellow hue. Dark-skinned women will find that a foundation color with a slight blue cast reflects their bronze beauty best. The easiest way to test a foundation is to apply a small amount and blend it into your jawline or forehead (not on your hands or wrists, which are a different color and texture). Then check out the effect in daylight, not just in the artificial light of the store.

Since we have varying skin types, here is how

Opposite: Subtle accents on lovely skin. *Right:* Foundation, a building block for a makeup regimen. *Top right:* Tyra Banks knows the secrets to great makeup.

TYRA BANKS
THE AIR ON PLANES IS USUALLY DRYING AND I TRAVEL A LOT. I CARRY A WATER ATOMIZER IN MY BAG AND GIVE MYSELF A COUPLE OF SPRITZES. I FOLLOW THIS UP WITH MOISTURIZER.

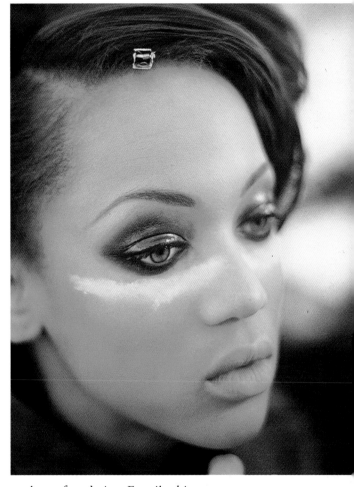

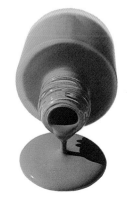

to choose foundation: For oily skin, use a water-based foundation. You'll probably need an oil-based or super-moisturizing foundation for dry skin. Combination skin does best with water-based products. Sensitive and acne-prone skin need a hypoallergenic, water-based foundation.

TRANSLUCENT POWDER Before applying blush, whisk or pat loose translucent powder all over your face with a powder puff or a large soft sable brush. This sets your makeup and

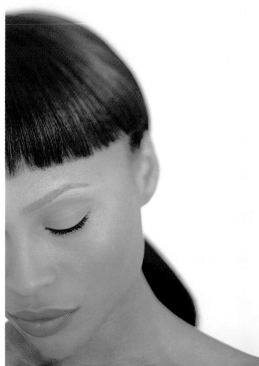

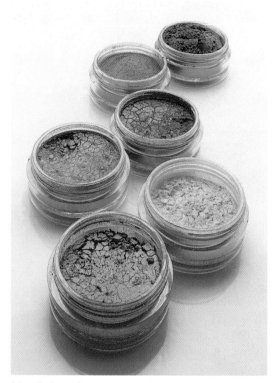

AALIYAH
THICKER BROWS MAKE MY LOOK, SO I MAKE SURE NOT TO ARCH THEM. I BRUSH THE BROW HAIRS DOWN, THEN CLIP EXCESS WITH SMALL SCISSORS. FOR A SOFTER LOOK I FILL THEM IN WITH POWDER.

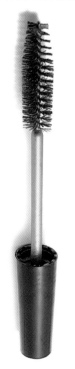

helps it to last longer. Powders for our skin usually come in three or four shades labeled Light or Sand, Medium or Clay, Dark or Bronze or something similar. Choose one in the same general family as your foundation. Women of color should stay away from any powders containing talc, the main offender in creating an "ashy" look to foundation.

BLUSH The most memorable cheeks are remembered for their bone structure, not the color. Blush colors are meant to create contours. They come in powder or creme and should be

Above: Soft makeup shades. *Right:* Replace mascara often. *Top right:* Colors give us many options. *Opposite:* A fresh, natural look.

blended up from the cheek or from the hairline to the cheek. You decide what works best for you. Bronzing powders meant for all-over facial application are also an excellent source of blushing beauty for women of color.

EYES

EYELINER Both pencils and liquid liners are now used to bring eyes center stage. How to pick and apply the right liner for you? Pencil liner gives a more natural look and is easier to use than liquid eyeliner, which requires a precise hand. Choose a creamy pencil, not a hard waxy one, or you may irritate

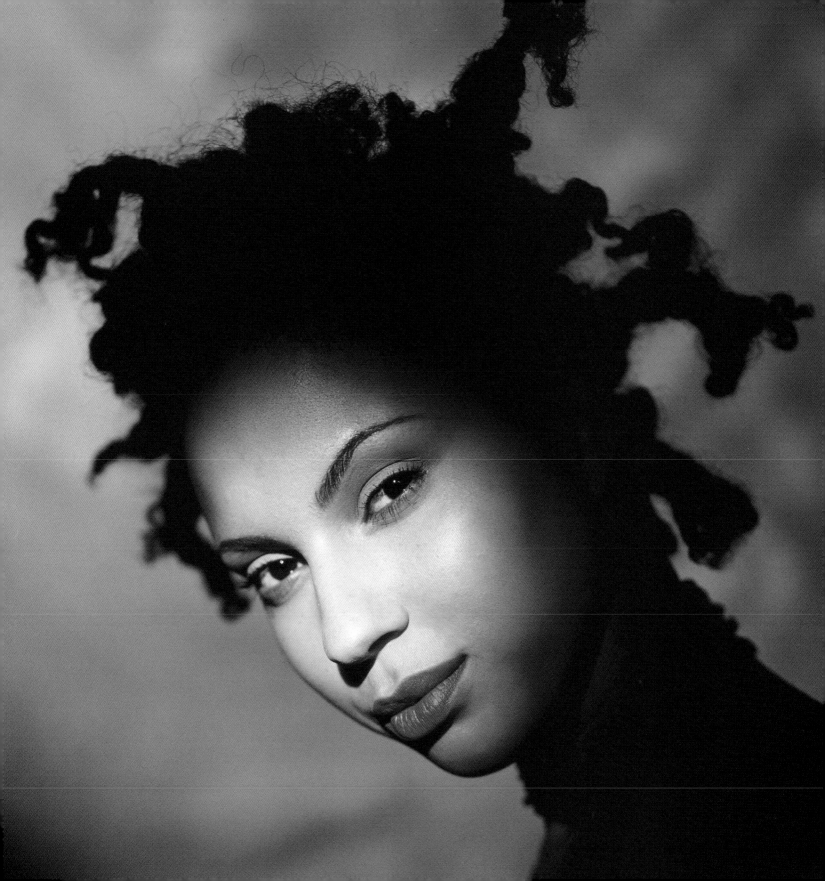

your eyes. To apply pencil liner: Starting at either corner of your eye, rest the tip of the pencil as close as possible to your lashes; keeping liner firm against lashes, draw a steady, smooth line across the lid. For liquid liner: Use a liquid formula with either a felt tip or a brush applicator; or turn your powder eye shadow into liner using a dampened angled brush.

MASCARA To create even more expressive eyes, curl your lashes before you apply mascara. Lash curlers are inexpensive and can be purchased at the drugstore. For the most fluttery pair of lashes, slowly work the wand from roots to ends. If clumping occurs, remove excess with an eyelash comb or toothbrush or dab

with your finger. A clean sweep: To remove mascara, moisten a flat cotton pad with a gentle eye-makeup remover and wipe away makeup. For hard-to-clean spots dampen a cotton swab with remover and dab. Remember, the more waterproof mascara is, the harder it will be to remove from your lashes. *Sanitary alert:* Replace mascara every three months and never share with anyone.

BROWS One season brows may be shapely, voluptuous, and curvy, the next they're thinner, refined, and elegant. Regardless of the trend of the moment, your brows set off and frame the beauty of your eyes. They form a natural line that shapes your face and eyes. Use that natural line as your guide when filling in

This page and opposite, left to right: a glossy glow; a creamy coat; the matte look; a sheer finish; a bit of shimmer and shine.

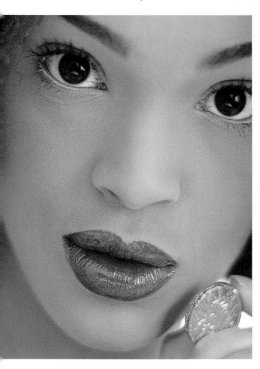
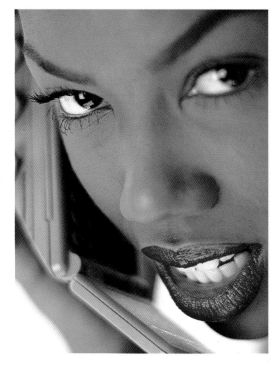
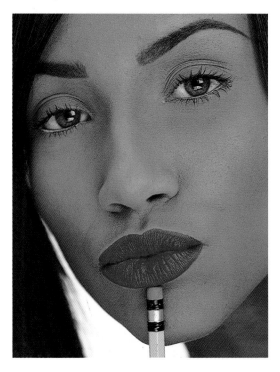

your brows. Tweezing: First, consider having your brows professionally waxed, then tackle growing-out strays with tweezers at home. Here's how: Clean and soften the area with a toner like witch hazel and a warm washcloth. Brush your eyebrows up to find the natural arch and look along the top of the brow for the peak. Start tweezing from underneath, pulling stray hairs. Make sure you don't pluck too many hairs from your brow's end point; this creates the too-plucked look.

FILLING IN BROWS Brows can be filled in with fine strokes of a pencil or eye shadows slightly lighter than your hair color. (Never use black even if your hair is black; it creates a hard, cartoonlike look.) Once you've

tweezed and filled in your brows, you can brush them in place.

LIPS

LIPSTICK A regular diet of certain matte lipsticks can leave your lips feeling a little raw. To keep lips soft, alternate your matte favorites with semi-matte or cream formulas that combine color with moisturizing ingredients such as aloe vera and shea butter. Some even provide sun protection and antioxidants that work to protect the lips from overexposure.

LIP PENCIL Outline your lips with a lip pencil that complements your lipstick color. They create great lip definition and help to prevent your lipstick from bleeding.

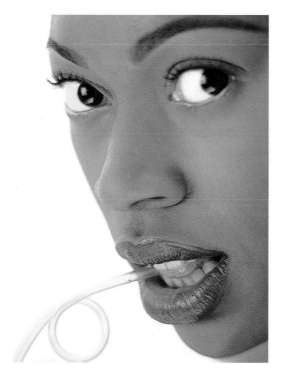

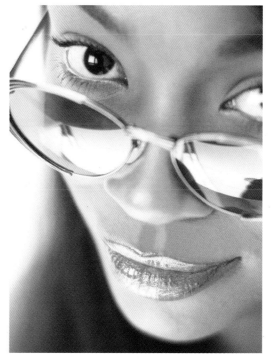

MAKING UP
IS EASY TO DO

Whether you're working the no-makeup look for an outdoor event, reporting to the office, or heading off to a Sisterella ball, you can achieve a great makeup look in no time. Here are three makeup cues you can pull off with the bat of a lash.

SPORTY/NATURAL Step 1: Opt for a light dusting of translucent powder or a tinted moisturizer. Step 2: Use either a brow pencil or powder to set brows, but not both. Or apply a simple application of mascara to your lashes. Step 3: Coat lips with a light application of lip gloss without lining lips first.

POWER MOVES Making up for the office can run the gamut from barely there to polished and professional. Step 1: Dab on concealer, liquid foundation, followed by powder. Step 2: Brush brows in an upward direction. Use an eye pencil or brow powder to fill in sparse areas. Step 3: Line lower lashes with a soft eye pencil. Coat lashes with mascara. Step 4: Apply coordinating blush, if desired. Step 5: Line lips using a coordinating lip pencil. Fill them in with matching lipstick.

GLAMOUR GIRL After putting on your base makeup, try one of these two sultry eye looks.

•THE SMOKY EYE Blend a light base shadow from brow bone to crease. To create the smoke effect, choose a deep-frosted or metallic shadow —charcoal grays, browns, greens, plums—and rim

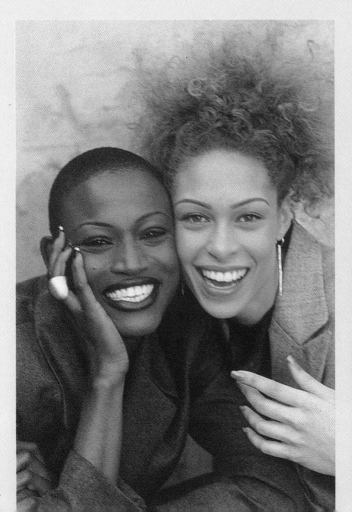

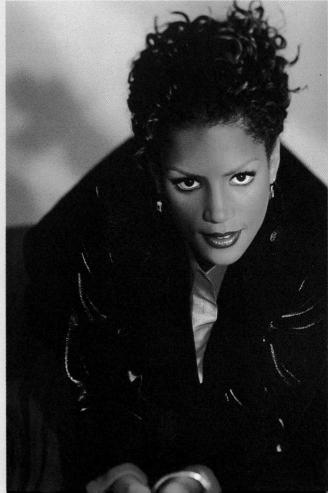

upper and lower lids. Use a sponge-tip applicator to line shadow on the top and bottom eyelids close to the lash and extend the shadow from the crease into the inner and outer corners of the eye. Gently blend shadow with a soft brush. Lastly, line outside rim of lower lashes with dark or matching eye pencil. Finish the look by sweeping the pencil's smudge tip over the line. Apply two coats of mascara.

• THE CAT EYE This glamorous "mod squad" look is always in style if you're the adventurous type (or at least feeling that way for a special occasion). Either sweep a light neutral shade all over the lid or a medium-tone shadow in the crease. Liquid liner gives a dramatic, precise effect for creating this look. First, pull lid taut with a fingertip. Resting the tip of the brush on your lashes, slowly stroke the brush from the inner corner to the outer corner of your eye, then apply mascara.

CAMERA AND PHOTOGRAPHY TIPS

Given the media-hyped society that we live in, chances are you'll get your fifteen minutes of fame. So whether you're slated for a television appearance, having professional photographs taken, or just making smiley faces in a videotape at your girlfriend's wedding, follow the tips of Juanita Dillard, owner of Imakeuup Makeup Artist, a line of cosmetics. Juanita reveals the biggest makeup mistakes sisters can make.

MISTAKE #1: TOO MUCH BLUSH! Tone down your too-bright blush with translucent powder.

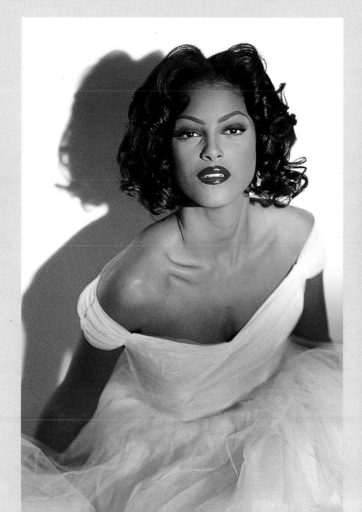

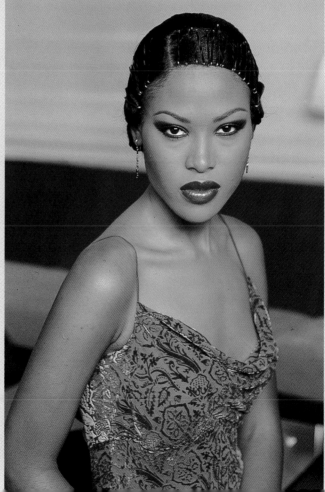

MISTAKE #2: EXCESSIVE LIP GLOSS.
Tissue it off and replace with a matte lipstick, then top it with a semi-gloss. Another culprit: yellow-gold frosted lipsticks. Wear a frosted bronze or brown-gold or brown-silver shade instead; they'll appear softer-looking and more natural.

MISTAKE #3: TOO MUCH SHINE. The camera zooms in on excess oil. Before you put on your foundation you'll need to apply an antishine primer, which blocks oil production before it reaches the skin's surface for hours at a stretch.

MISTAKE #4: TOO MUCH EYE SHADOW.
Your best bet is to stick with a neutral palette of browns, tans, and chestnuts. Color under the brow bone; the darkest color in the crease, the medium shade on the lids above the lash line.

Below left: Soft neutral shades give the bride a fresh, beautiful look. *Opposite:* Monica, recording artist.

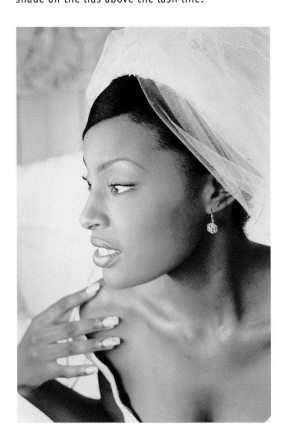

THE BEAUTY BAR

"Don't use eye or blush brushes in department stores. Studies have shown they're magnets for a multitude of bacteria problems. To try an eye shadow or blush shade, use a Q-tip or cotton ball, respectively. Ask the sales clerk for a pencil sharpener and sharpen all eye and lip pencils before trying them. Try a lipstick shade by wiping a tester on the back of your hand. Don't use mascara unless it has been wiped with an antibacterial spray." —Robin Emtage, makeup artist

"Makeup for your wedding day should be serene, opulent, and traditional. Stick to brown, gray, and taupe eye shadows in the traditional tricolor contour: the lightest shade right under brow bone; the darkest in the crease and a medium tone on lids. And for groom-proof kisses, cover lips with foundation first, then a dusting of translucent powder. Follow with lip liner, matte lipstick, then more powder. Blot lips with tissue then apply lipstick once again." —Lanier Long, makeup artist

"Every woman of color has a natural eye shadow on her lids. Take petroleum jelly or baby oil and rub it on the entire lid to make it look like you're wearing makeup!" —Nzingha, makeup artist

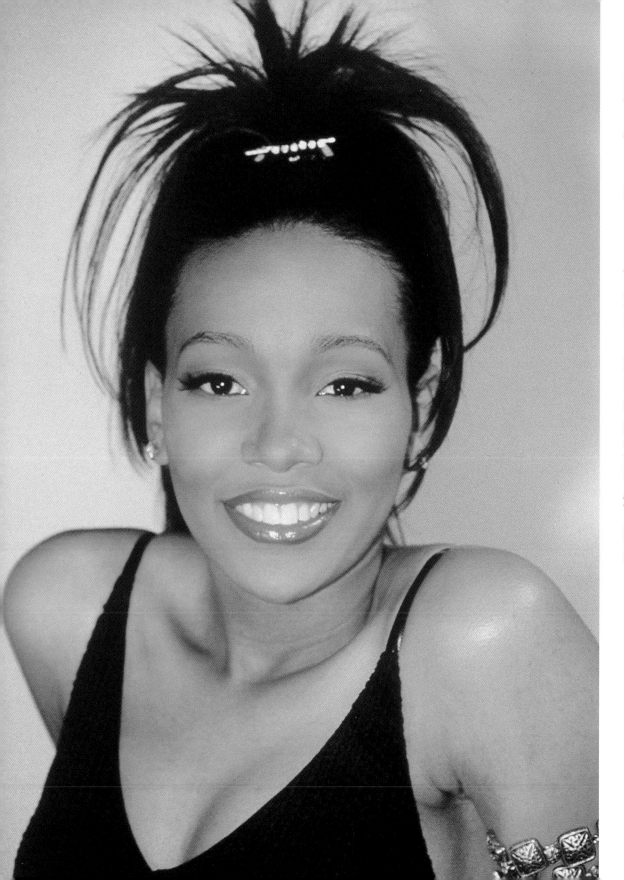

MONICA
TO CREATE
A MORE
NATURAL
LOOK ON MY
CHEEKS I
DON'T USE
BLUSH.
INSTEAD, I
TAKE TWO
SHADES OF
PRESSED
POWDER—
ONE THAT IS
MY SKIN
COLOR; THE
OTHER
SLIGHTLY
DARKER—
AND BRUSH
THEM ON MY
CHEEKS LIKE
BLUSH.

THE MAKEOVERS

Facial skin is delicate. When it erupts it's difficult to know how to treat such outbreaks, and so many times what we do hurts more than it helps. *Essence* wanted to know the real deal on how to combat a rebellious epidermis, so we sent three sisters who were having problems with their skin to the experts to help figure things out and restore their skin to its natural beauty.

Tareeka

Tareeka ran into trouble by committing a beauty no-no: shaving her face. As a result, her skin suffered from painful ingrown hairs, especially on her chin and neck, dark discolorations, and a case of mild acne with plenty of pimples. Because her condition was serious but confined only to the top layer of skin, *Essence* sent Tareeka to Irma Denson, veteran skin-care expert and owner of the Irma Denson Skin Care Salon and Day Spa in New York City.

On her first visit, Irma gave Tareeka a soothing deep-cleansing facial to relax the skin and treat the acne. By using a benzol peroxide/alpha hydroxy peel followed by a steaming session, Irma was able to work the skin and gently remove the dirt, whiteheads and

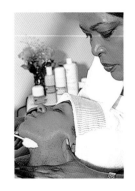

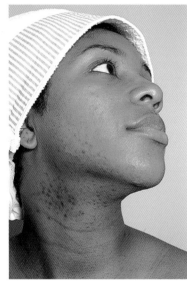

Top and above: Before. *Opposite:* Tareeka's healthy glow is renewed through aesthetician Irma Denson's care. **Tareeka is not wearing foundation in this photograph.**

blackheads, and toxins from Tareeka's face. Irma then removed all of Tareeka's facial hair through waxing. Many times waxing is better than tweezing, which can break the hair and leave the follicle embedded in the skin.

Tareeka was quickly on the road to recovery. During her second visit, Irma used an exfoliant with a mild alcohol base to open Tareeka's follicles and keep the hair from turning in again, while Tareeka began a new beauty regimen at home. She kept her face clean with a mild azulene cleanser mixed with a facial shampoo, and Irma also gave her a toner, an aloe cream, and a strawberry mask to balance her oily T-zone with drier parts of her face. To even out her skin tone, Tareeka used a bleaching cream on the dark areas each night, and a sunblock during the day to protect her face's sensitive areas.

By her third trip to Irma Denson's spa, Tareeka's skin had cleared up and the scarring left behind by shaving was already beginning to fade. She continued to see Irma for weekly facials and waxing treatments every two weeks, but the biggest reason for Tareeka's return to radiance was her enthusiastic commitment to taking care of her face on a daily basis, using the knowledge she learned from Irma. After three months, her face had regained its clarity and gentle glow.

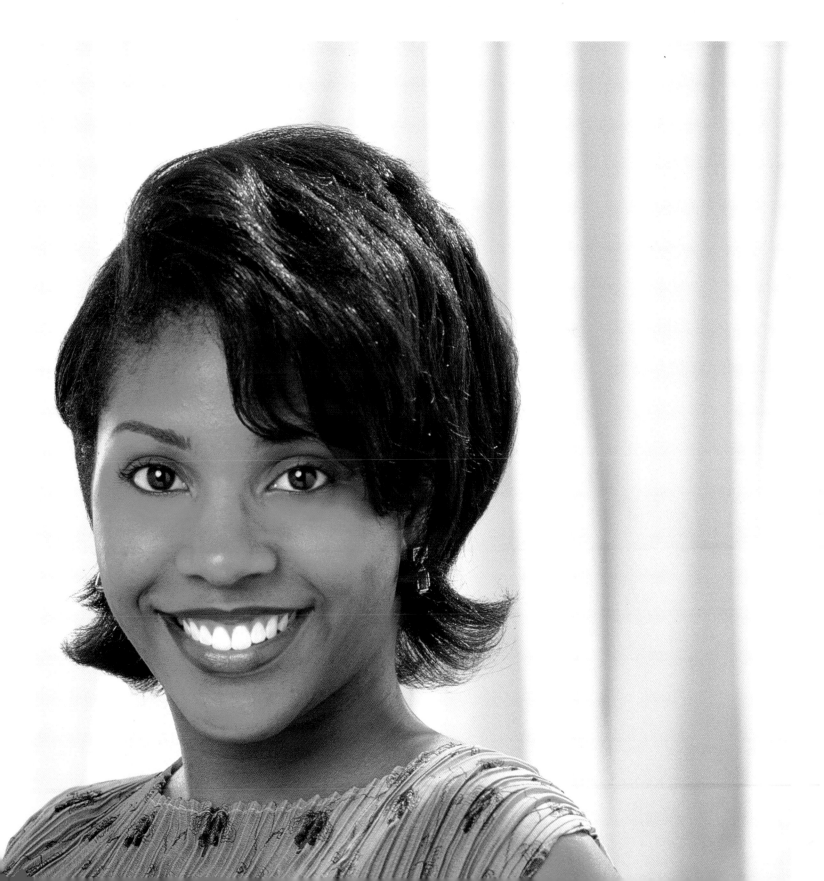

Michele

Some Black women develop skin problems that need a medical doctor's attention. When Michele met with Dr. Deborah A. Simmons, the noted New York City dermatologist who is expert in treating Black skin, Dr. Simmons diagnosed her as having dermatosis papulosa nigra (DPN), a condition usually affecting sisters in their late thirties and early forties. DPN is recognized by black, bumpy skin growths on the face. These hereditary bumps aren't cancerous, but they can itch and be unsightly. Michele also had a case of mild acne, and skin tags on her neck—raised flaps of skin that can itch as well.

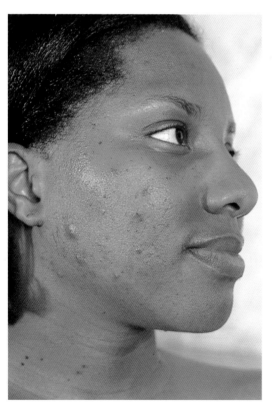

Dr. Simmons easily removed the skin tags with surgical scissors after the skin was numbed with a local anesthetic. She had Michele treat the acne with twice-daily applications of a benzoyl peroxide/erythromycin gel. Getting rid of the DPN was more complicated. Dr. Simmons dealt with the bumps (also known as "papules") through a process called "electrodesiccation." Electrodesiccation uses a device that passes a low-grade electric current through the skin to "burn off" the papules. This procedure runs the risk of leaving areas of light or dark spots of discoloration on some Black skin so it's important to see a dermatologist who's very well trained in using the process.

Electrodesiccation worked for Michele. The papules were removed after two treatment sessions, leaving no signs of scarring or discoloration on her skin several weeks later. New DPN lesions may develop over time, so Dr. Simmons recommended that Michele have follow-up treatments once or twice a year.

Left: Before. *Opposite:* **Michele is photographed without foundation** after Dr. Simmons's successful treatment.

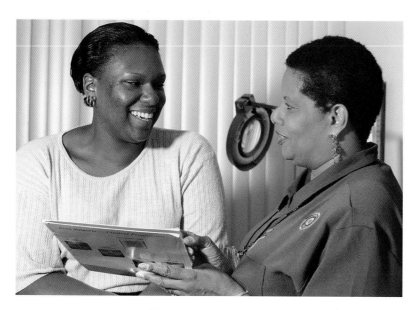

Above: Before. *Opposite:* **Tracey is photographed with no foundation** after two months under Dr. Simmons's care.

Tracey

Dr. Simmons also treated Tracey, a sister with moderate to severe acne on her face and neck. The acne was made worse by seborrheic dermatitis, an overgrowth of yeast on the scalp resulting in an itchy, flaky, serious dandruff. Dermatitis contributes to the acne because the buildup of oil and grease on the scalp leads to excess oil on the face.

A severe case of acne often needs to be treated with oral antibiotics, but Dr. Simmons told Tracey that her face's condition would improve by simply washing her hair more often. Like many sisters with relaxers, Tracey only washed her hair every two or three weeks, and tried to keep her head moisturized with too much oil. Washing her hair once a week kept her skin cleaner, and she used a lighter, glycerin-based hair dressing sparingly when her hair needed a little extra moisture and sheen.

The more frequent washings immediately improved Tracey's complexion. Dr. Simmons also had her use three topical agents for even greater gains in facial freshness: a mild astringent twice a day after washing to reduce dirt and oil; an antibiotic gel twice daily to reduce bacteria; and a tretinoin formula to use at night for acne pimples and discolorations.

After one month of treatment Dr. Simmons noted an improvement in Tracey's skin. She had fewer whiteheads and blackheads, less oil on her face, and the acne discolorations had lightened. After two months, her face had almost cleared up completely and Tracey was back to having beautiful, healthy skin.

A NOTE OF CAUTION: *Always follow your physician's guidelines when using antibiotics and other drugs or chemicals on your face. Overuse can result in serious and/or long-term damage to the skin. Pregnant women or women contemplating pregnancy should consult their doctor before undertaking any course of treatment.*

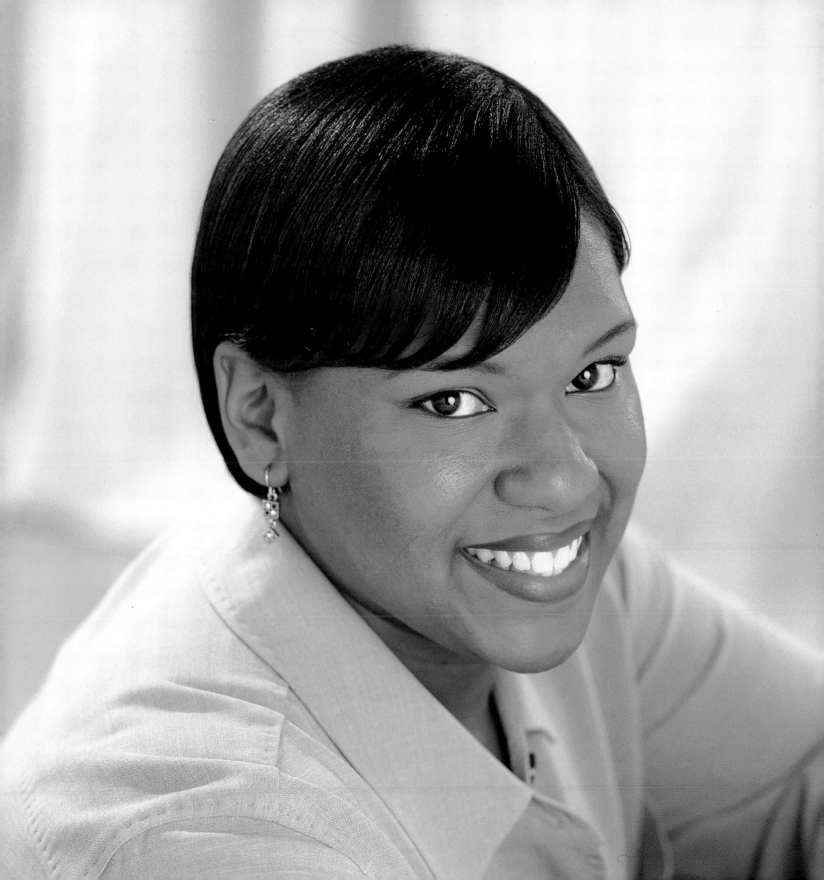

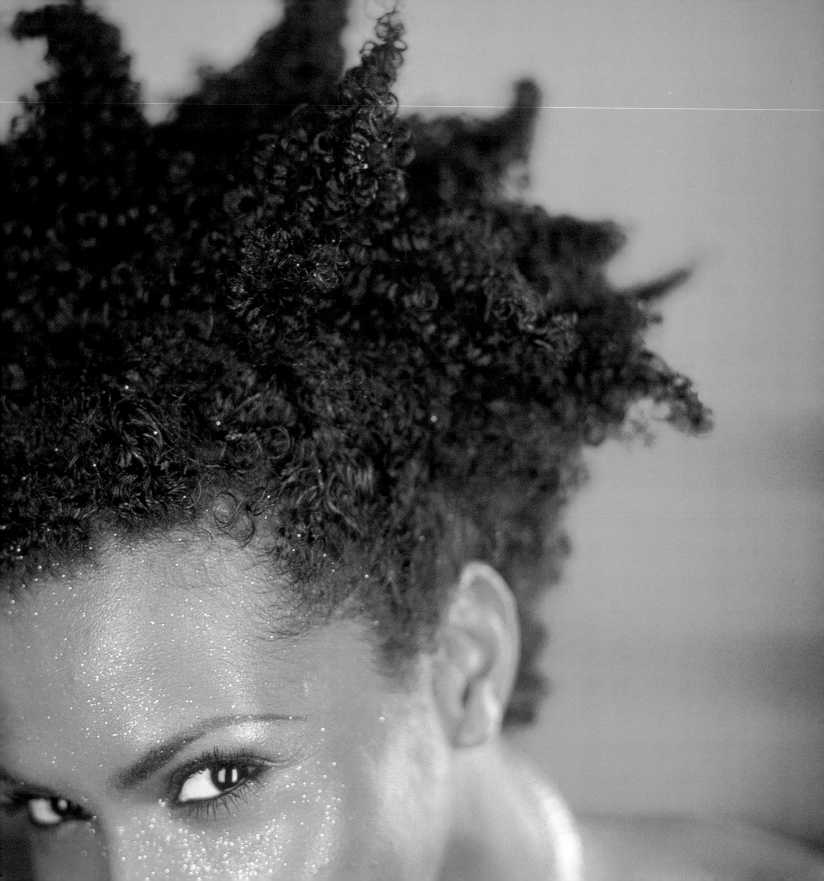

2 CELEBRATING OUR HAIR

WHETHER IT IS THE SUPER-BAD, SUPER-FLY, SUPER-SIZED AFRO; Motherland-inspired, intricately woven braids; divinely inspired locks; or a fiercely angled short cut, we are known for our ever-changing hair. Black women possess the most versatile hair on earth, and boy, do we work it! We can sculpt, mold, curl, and shape our hair into any style imaginable. Our hair textures come in a glorious range of shapes from poker straight, to softly waved, to gravity-defying kinky.

Our hair and hair-styling methods telegraph volumes about our culture. Our creativity is depicted for posterity in the funereal art of the royal ancient Egyptians as finely woven braids and spiral curls dressed in lotus blossoms and lapis. That creative spirit traveled with our ancestors from

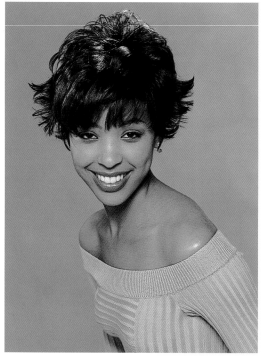

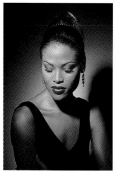

Left: A short flip. *Above:* Pure elegance, hair has a French roll in back and a head band at the crown. *Right:* Traditional styles of the Motherland are revisited with Bantu knots. *Opposite:* Dual-tone effects captivate in coil-set hair.

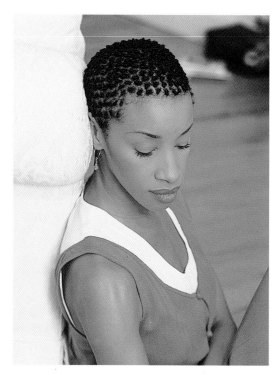

Africa to the shores of the Americas. Our inventiveness is carried out by the Himba women of modern Namibia, who lengthen their hair with twists of sheep's wool and then set it in place with a mixture of mud, fat, and ochre. There are a wealth of examples. Yes, folks all over are amazed by our resourcefulness, artistry, and sense of beauty.

When we are not turning style on its ear, our hair brings us together and fosters lasting communal bonds. Many of our earliest memories revolve around sitting in between Mommy's or Grandma's knees getting our hair greased, combed, and braided. Many of us remember the rites of passage of our first press and curl for our elementary school pictures or the womanly mystery of the beauty salon.

There is power in our tightly curled mane. The return to natural in the early seventies made the Afro a political statement and a defiant declaration of our unaltered bold Black beauty. Our richly textured hair is part of a profound legacy and the antithesis of the wrongheaded antiquated notions of "good hair" versus "bad hair." Hair this powerful can only be good!

Our crowning glory is both an expression of personal style and a reminder of a proud past. No matter how you wear it, you want it to be at its best: healthy and flattering to you. You want to treat your hair with love, because hair, like anything else, responds to nurturing and attention.

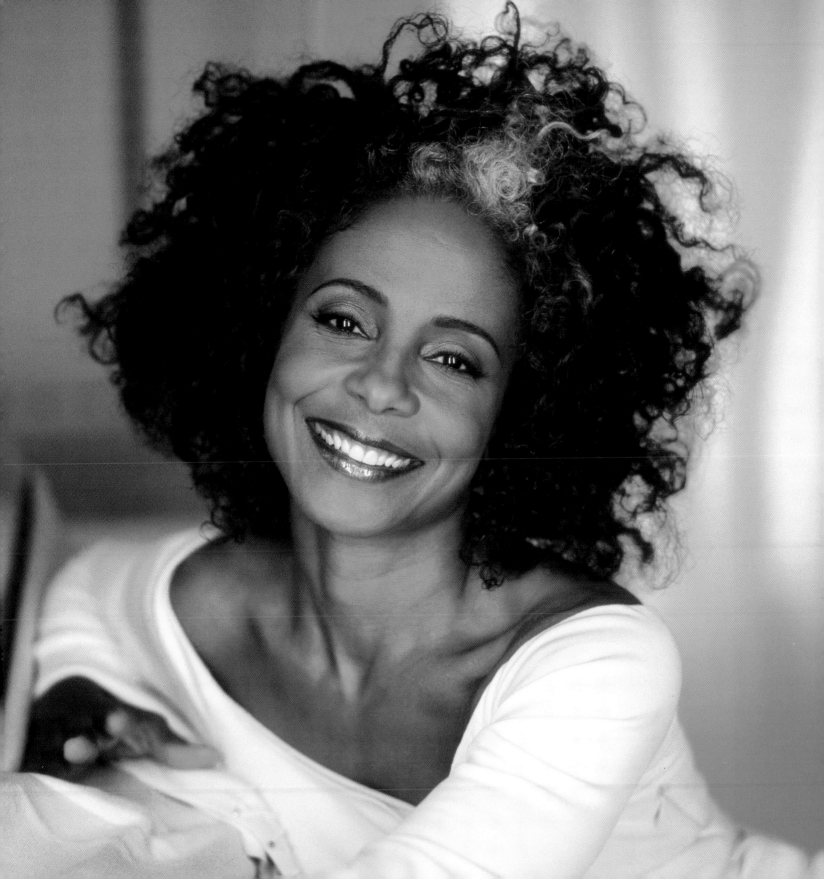

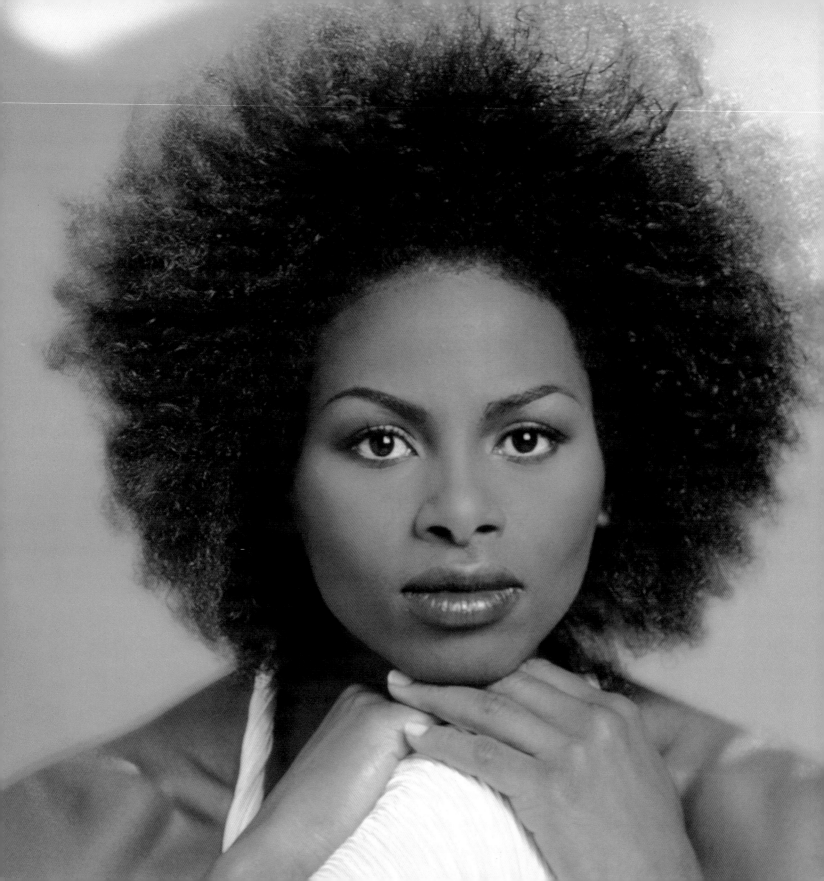

ASSESS YOUR TRESSES

Get to know your hair's natural state. Look at it closely, touch it. Not only will you enjoy the sensual pleasures, but you will also gain a sense of how healthy it is. Before you braid, weave, or retouch your hair, try these simple steps as a test to tell you more about your hair's structure and condition.

Texture

This refers to three elements: curl configuration, or whether the hair is straight, wavy, curly, or extremely curly; diameter of the hair, or the size of the individual strands; and the feel of the hair, or whether the hair is hard or soft, smooth or wiry to the touch.

To test for texture:

• Pull out a strand of your hair.

• Place your index finger and thumb on the strand, and slide them up and down along its length.

• If the strand of hair feels hard and wiry and looks thick, then it is most likely "coarse." If it feels soft and smooth and looks thin, then it is probably "fine." Your hair can also be hard and thin or soft and thick.

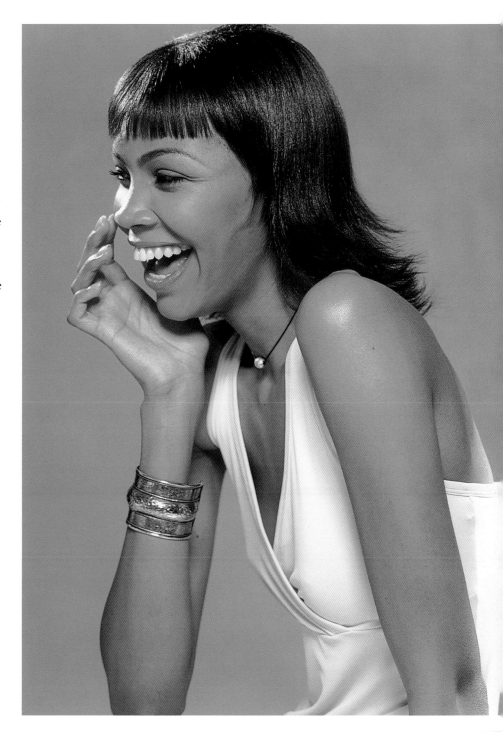

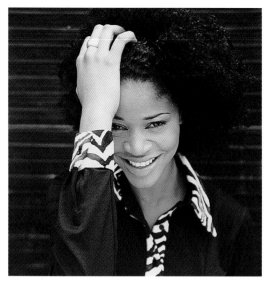

Porosity

Hair needs moisture to survive and thrive. Porosity refers to the hair's ability to absorb moisture or chemicals, and is determined by the diameter of the strand (thick, medium, or fine).

To test for porosity:

• Lift the hair from the scalp with one hand, and push the strands downward toward the scalp with the other hand, as though teasing.

• If the hair bunches up as it is teased, it is very porous. If the hair bunches up somewhat, it is normal. If the hair bunches up a little, or not at all, it is resistant.

Thick hair strands do not absorb as much moisture as fine or relaxed hair strands, which tend to be more porous. The more porous your hair is the more vulnerable it is to damage from chemicals, and because it's absorbent it "receives" chemical treatments more quickly and requires less time for dyes and relaxers to take effect.

Elasticity

Elasticity refers to the hair's ability to stretch and return to its original size and shape— without breaking! Hair with normal elasticity is springy and shiny in appearance, and can stretch about one-fifth of its length when dry and one-half its length when wet.

To test for elasticity:

• Select a hair strand and hold it between the index fingers and thumbs of both hands.

• Gently pull the strand and note its elasticity.

• If it stretches and returns to its original length, your hair's elasticity is good. If it breaks, its elasticity is poor. Poor elasticity is the first clue that you are overdoing any chemical or heat applications including relaxers, color treatments, curly permanents, and blow-drying.

HAIR STRUCTURE

Although we tend to think of our hair as an outlet of personal expression, the original purpose of hair was quite basic: It covers the head to cushion you from blows, and it keeps your head warm in cold weather and cool under the heat of the sun. And even though our hair is quite versatile, we must keep in mind that it is delicate as well.

Straight or curly, the basic structure of hair is the same. Hair is composed of a hard chemi-

Opposite: Spiral coils with a lush textured finish.

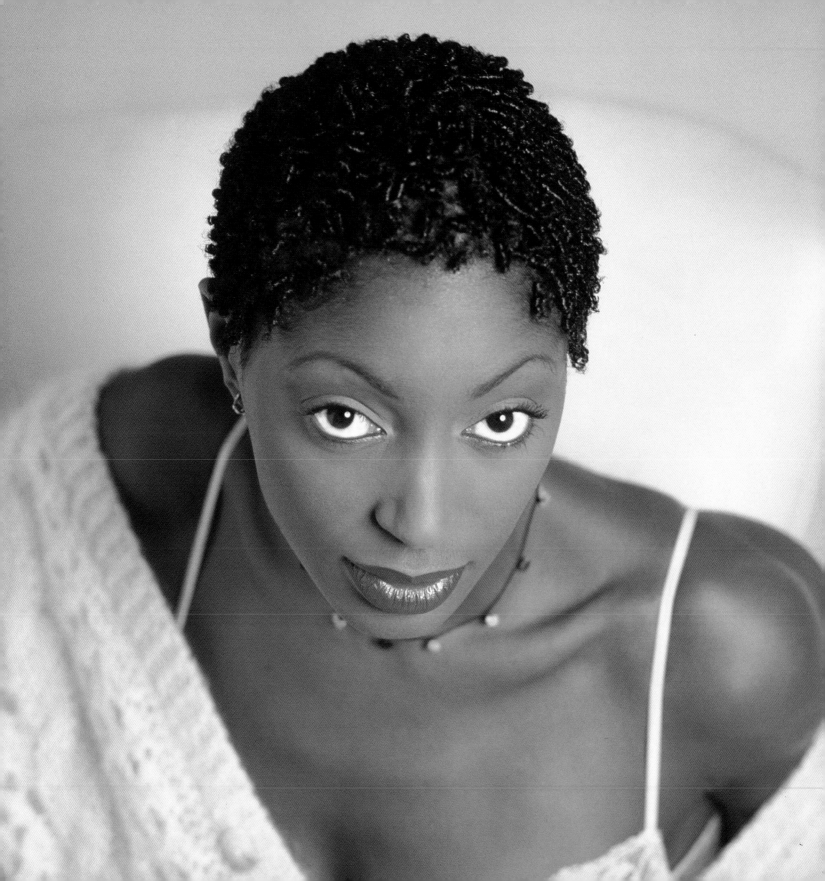

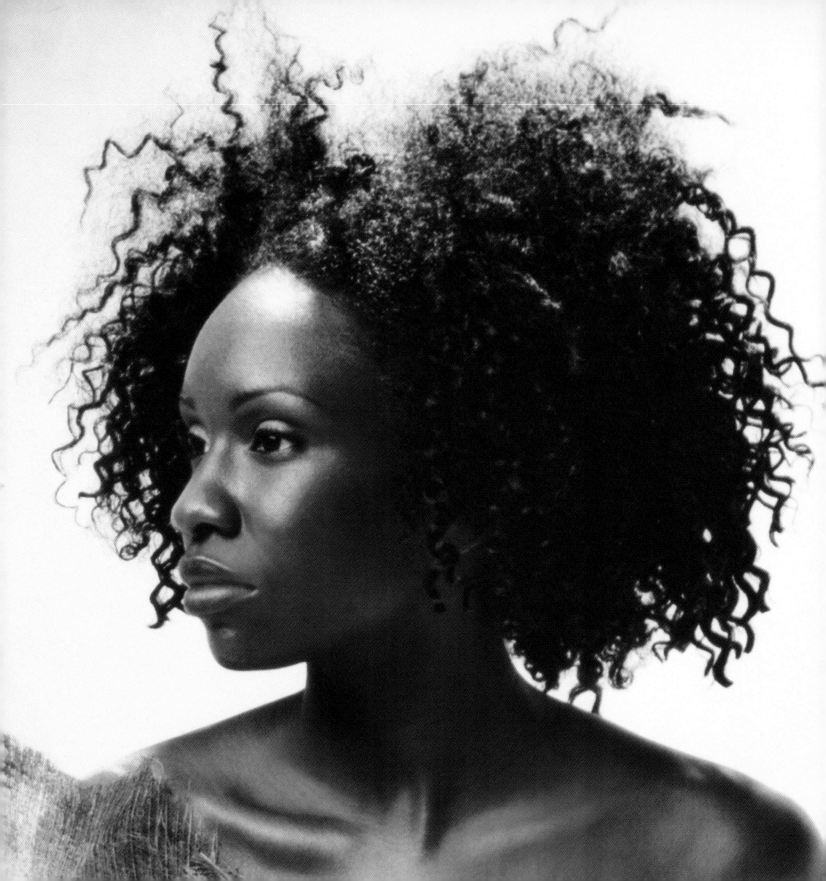

cal substance called keratin, a sulfur-rich protein that provides the hair with strength and is resistant to being dissolved (think of all the chemicals we use on it). The part of the hair that grows above the scalp (and is what we generally concern ourselves with) is the hair shaft or strand. Each strand of hair comes out of a tiny tubelike pit in the skin called a follicle, at the base of which is the papilla, the hair's source for blood, oxygen, nutrients, and new cells. As the cells in the papilla multiply to become an individual hair, they arrange themselves into three separate layers: the cuticle, the cortex, and the medulla.

As the outermost layer of the hair shaft, the cuticle is composed of transparent, overlapping cells resembling the scales of a fish. It is the cuticle that protects against excessive moisture loss while at the same time preventing chemicals from penetrating into the core of the hair. Really curly or kinky hair has fewer cuticle layers than straighter hair, so it has less protection from the damage we inflict upon it. Each time you go for a touch-up, or use a curling iron or blow dryer, you destroy a cuticle layer and lose much-needed moisture. Beneath the cuticle lies the cortex, which contains the pigment that gives hair its color. The innermost portion of the hair is the medulla, a small core of cells that runs the length of the hair shaft. This loose arrangement of cells is sensitive and can be destroyed by chemicals and physical damage.

One of the biggest myths about super-curly

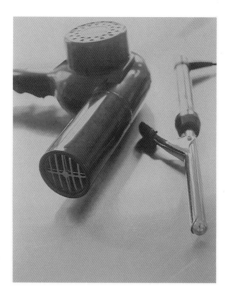

Opposite: Hair this powerful can only be good! *Above:* Quality hair care means using the right tools.

or kinky hair is that it doesn't grow. Not true! Hair growth is a constant process for everybody. The average rate of growth is one half inch per month and up to six or eight inches a year. The average head has 120,000 strands of hair, and we normally lose from 50 to 100 hairs daily, so over time the mane thins out as we age. But why is the no-growth myth so prevalent in the community? Quite simply, chemicals, heat implements, and overuse of tools, even simply combing and brushing, cause hair to break. And hair growth is not as noticeable on tightly curled hair, thus we never seem to gain any appreciable length.

In our fast-paced, service-oriented society, too many of us just blindly turn our treasured tresses over to someone else. Every woman needs to know her hair type, what healthy hair looks and feels like, and she should have a general sense of what her hair can and cannot do.

We should share this information with our stylists, and try to create a true partnership in maintaining healthy hair. How many of us spent too many years insisting on a hairstyle that looked best with one type of hair while we had another? Just think of the time you could have saved by adopting a style that enhanced your hair's natural strengths instead of slink-

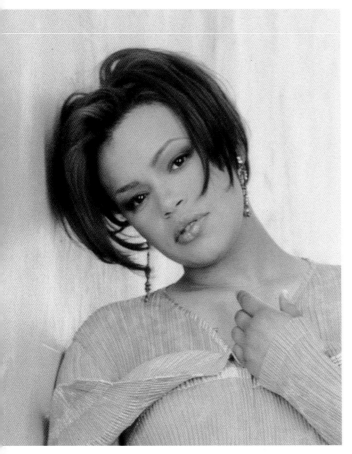

Above: Faith Evans, singer.

ing out of the chair, vaguely disappointed. Often we go into the salon with a picture or an image of what we want our hair to look like, without taking into account that our type of hair and its health cannot yield that result.

Understanding your hair type and regularly assessing it will not only make you aware of the treatments and the styles that are best for you, it can also serve as an early indicator of your own health. Many illnesses affecting the rest of the body show warning signs in the hair.

GET DOWN TO BASICS

It cannot be stressed enough how delicate some of our hair is. Chemicals, heat, mechanical manipulation (combing and brushing), even the environment affects our precious strands. Thus, healthy, great-looking hair is an ongoing quest that requires more than a part-time interest. It all begins with a hair-care regimen. The regimen does not have to be rigorous and all-consuming, but it should consist of a good cut, regular trims and maintenance, proper use of tools, quality products, and an affirming attitude toward your mane. Also, don't overlook the importance of a good diet, one that is rich in nutrients—found in fish, beans, poultry, fruit, veggies, and vitamin B complex.

The Wash Cycle

A quick look through any sister's bathroom is bound to uncover several bottles of half-used shampoo. Among the ruins are the cleansers that promised to do everything but pay your rent, and those formulated for a specific (but wrong for you) hair type. All that is really needed is a cleanser that breaks down dirt, oil, and product buildup, and can easily wash them away. As a rule of thumb, we should wash our hair at least once a week with a

SHAMPOO GLOSSARY

Here is a listing of various types of popular shampoos and how they benefit your hair.

CLARIFYING Deep-cleanser usually with concentrated detergents designed to remove waxy buildup from styling products and metallic deposits from water. Good for swimmers; however, because of heavy detergents, it s a limited-use product.

COLOR-ENHANCING A gentle cleansing shampoo with silicone and color protectors that help keep color intact.

CONDITIONING Has beneficial ingredients panthenol, keratin proteins, amino acids that help normalize pH level.

DETANGLING With ingredients such as dimethicone, to soften hair cuticle.

EXTRA-BODY Contains thickeners and/or bonding ingredients that expand fine hair and give the appearance of fuller hair.

MEDICATED Many contain selenium sulfide, pyrithone zinc, or coal tar; advisable for dandruff control and/or itchy, tingling scalp.

MOISTURIZING Has humectants, which pull moisture from the air, and other moisture-giving ingredients.

PROTEIN Uses protein from a variety of sources wheat, soy, keratin that bond with hair and smooth the outer layer of the hair.

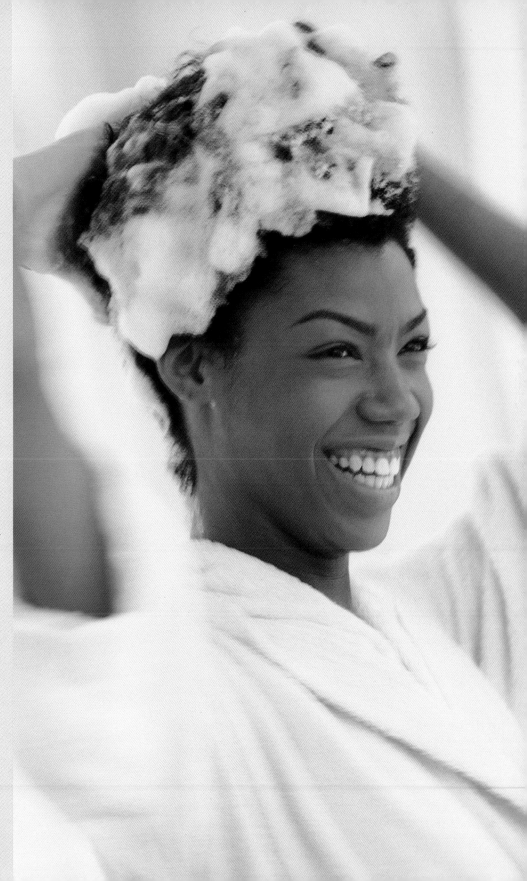

shampoo that is right for our own hair needs.

What should we consider when selecting a shampoo? Get one that contains detanglers to eliminate pulling and tugging, which are particularly abusive to the curly texture of our hair. Read labels to learn the pH level, or the acid/alkaline content. Hair's normal pH is 4.5 to 5.5. Shampoo with a pH of 4.5 to 5.5 is great for dry and damaged hair because it shrinks the cuticle and makes the hair shaft stronger and shinier. Anything lower is too acidic and will harden the hair. Anything higher will act as an alkali and soften the hair. Look for a formula with moisturizers and antistatic ingredients to smooth hair, eliminate flyaways, and help avoid split ends. Another safe bet is protein shampoos to strengthen and build up elasticity in the hair shaft. Avoid clear shampoos, which generally signal more detergent than conditioners; good conditioning shampoos tend to be creamy and pearlized.

For proper shampooing follow these steps. Gently brush hair to loosen dandruff, product buildup, and stray hairs. Then wet hair with warm water. Using no more than a teaspoon of shampoo gently work it into the scalp and massage through the hair to achieve a lather. Rinse thoroughly and repeat the process. Let go of the old-time adage about squeaky clean hair. The truth is that squeaky hair means you've stripped your hair of its natural oils.

THE CONDITIONING PROCESS

Make the term *conditioning* your mantra. This is the most important process in caring for our hair, whether it is natural, relaxed, color-treated, or heat-treated. A conditioner can strengthen damaged hair and maintain healthy hair. Conditioners were created to restore moisture, strength, body, and manageability to the hair. In addition, conditioning also helps flatten and smooth the cuticle of each strand and promotes shine.

While the conditioner is hair's number one first-aid tool, it can only restore the appearance of the hair. A conditioner is not a miracle cure. It will bind a split end, but keep in mind that the ends are still split and damaged. Nothing is going to heal the hair except a good snip!

Below: A carefree pixie cut. *Opposite:* Nancy Wilson, jazz stylist.

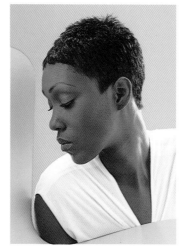

Conditioning your hair once a week with either a leave-in or wash-out conditioner is a must. Chemically treated hair (relaxed or colored) should receive a deep conditioning treatment once a month. If hair is really damaged, the best course is to alternate between a moisturizing conditioner and a protein conditioner to boost weak strands.

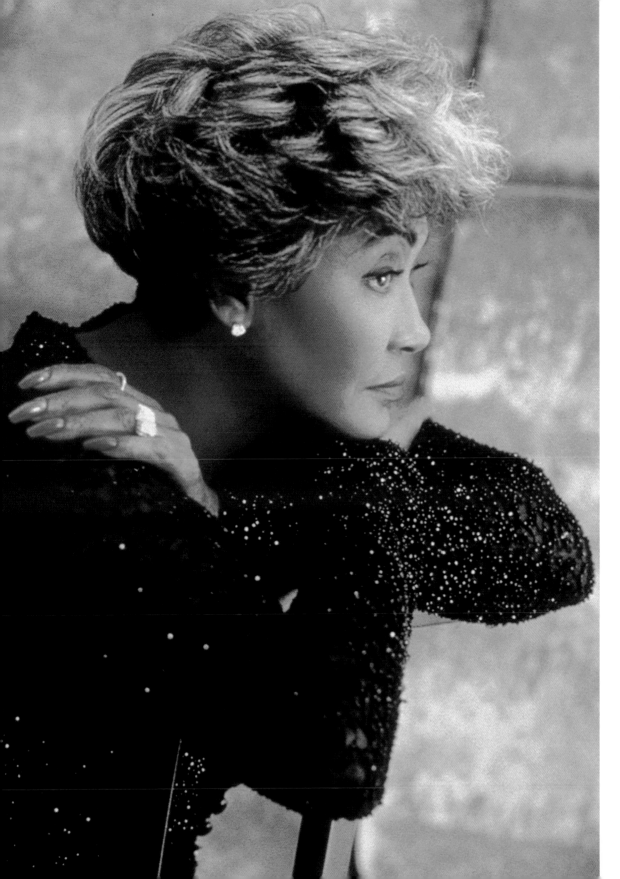

NANCY WILSON I LOVE MY GRAY HAIR AND TREAT IT GENTLY BY KEEPING IT MOISTURIZED. I NEVER USE CURLING IRONS; HEAT TURNS GRAY HAIR YELLOW.

CONDITIONER GLOSSARY

Here's the 411 you should know on the categories of conditioners.

INSTANT OR WASH-OUT Coats the surface of the hair with protein and oil and restores moisture, increases the diameter of each strand, flattens cuticle, thus hair appears fuller and shiny. Instant conditioners also protect the hair from blow-drying, sun exposure, and chemical processes.

LEAVE-IN Styling product/conditioning combo has a light, watery consistency that infuses hair with moisture and offers a shiny finish. It can be used daily.

RECONSTRUCTIVE/DEEP Protein-based conditioners are designed to penetrate the cuticle and bolster the cortex. These products restore moisture and give protection to the hair shaft making it less frayed and brittle. They provide a source of moisture and are made specifically for dry and damaged hair. This type of conditioner is usually left on the hair for twenty to thirty minutes (often with a heating cap or the dryer), then rinsed out.

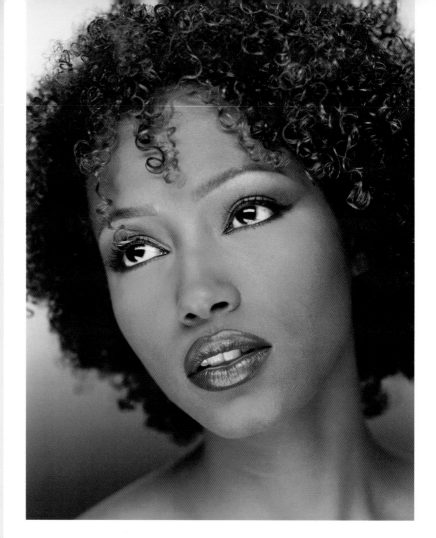

HAIR TOOLS

Here is what to have on hand to help you care for your hair in the kindest fashion.

WIDE-TOOTHED COMB Whether your hair is natural or relaxed, thin or fine, everyone needs a wide-toothed comb because of the ease in which it detangles our hair. Make sure the comb is made of rubber or tortoiseshell because those materials are gentle to the hair. Plastic combs tend to cut and split hair strands.

NATURAL-HAIR BRISTLE BRUSH Look for either natural- or boar-hair bristles when select-

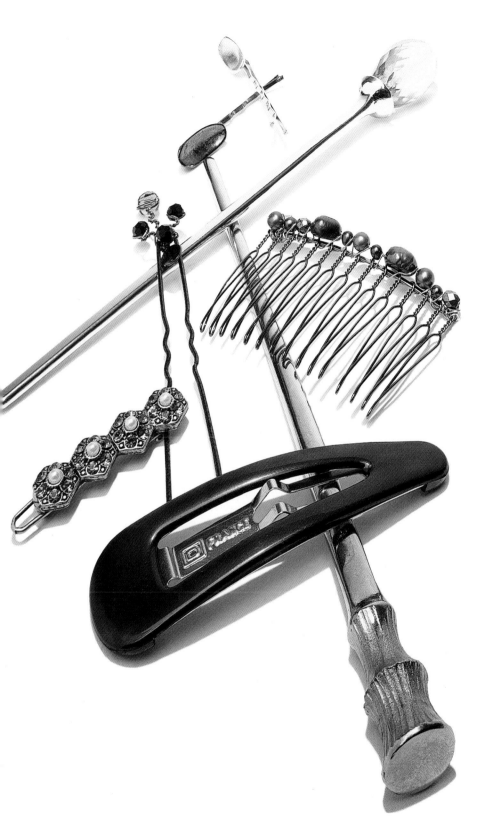

ing a brush. Natural bristles tenderly smooth hair, distribute natural oils from the scalp to the hair shaft, and stimulate the scalp.

ROLLERS Mesh and metallic rollers work best for a long-lasting set. Mesh rollers used with end papers and hairpins are great because they create tension that helps retain the shape the hair dries in. Jumbo metallic rollers give medium to long relaxed hair body and bounce and are easier to use.

BLOW-DRYER Use for quick drying and styling. The experts agree that it's a time-saving tool but warn that at 1200 watts, dryers have sufficient wattage to get hair straight without frying it, and that appliances should be kept moving and ten to twelve inches away from your hair. Alternate with the hood dryer.

CURLING IRON Use for quick curls and to further smooth hair. Look for a thermostatically controlled iron to avoid burning hair. And use only on clean hair with a moisture cream to buffer your ends from the heat.

HOOD DRYER Hands down, the healthiest way to dry your hair. The indirect heat will seal moisture in for supple strands.

SILK SCARVES AND SATIN BONNETS Wrap hair at night before bedtime to maintain your hairstyle. Silk or satin fabric protects hair from friction and breakage that results from using cotton pillowcases.

BOBBY PINS AND HAIRPINS They offer control in shaping the hair. Make sure that both have the rubber tips to avoid splitting the hair and scratching the scalp.

SHOWER CAP Keeps hair from getting wet in the shower; when used with a conditioner, it acts as a mini-heating cap by trapping body heat.

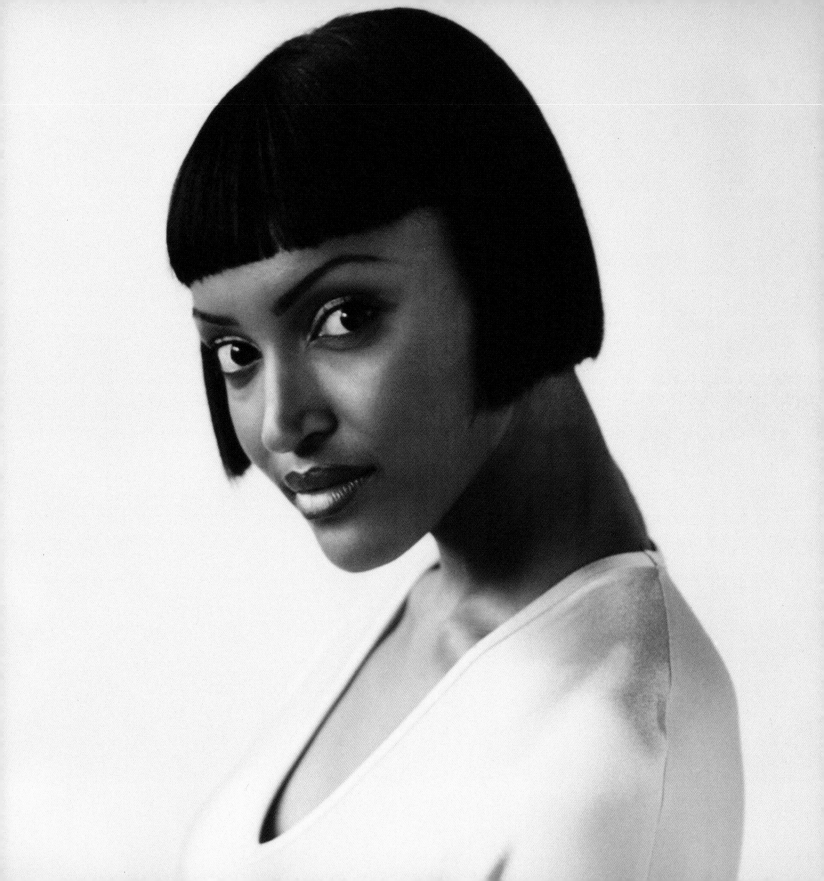

STRAIGHT TALK

CARE OF RELAXED HAIR

Over 75 percent of us sport relaxed hair. The ease of styling and the various sleek looks give the relaxer an undeniable lure. What exactly does a relaxer do? In short, the active ingredient—either sodium hydroxide (lye) or calcium hydroxide (*no-lye* is the term, but quite frankly it is still lye)—breaks down the hydrogen and sulfide bonds that give the hair its shape. The relaxer is then combed through and pulled straight.

It is left on the hair for a specific amount of time (the average is eight minutes) depending on the strength of the hair, tightness of the curl pattern, and how straight you want your hair to be. Now the chemical is rearranging the hair bonds in a straighter fashion. Then the relaxer is rinsed off and the hair is washed with a neutralizing shampoo to stop the relaxing process and to restore the hair's pH balance. After the neutralizer is washed out, a conditioner is applied. The relaxed look is maintained by touching up the hair's new growth every six to eight weeks.

Unfortunately, a relaxer's potent chemicals heighten the risk of damage and breakage to the hair. Also the best relaxer and application will still leave hair in a fragile, weakened state.

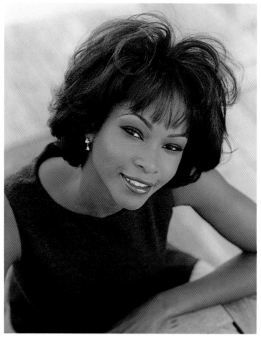

In order to keep the margin of error to a minimum, leave the relaxing process to a professional stylist.

CARE OF RELAXED HAIR Wash hair once a week with a shampoo specifically for chemically treated hair. Follow with a conditioner.

If your hair is in good shape, go for an instant conditioner and once every three weeks treat it with hot oil or a deep conditioner. Damaged hair should alternate between a moisturizing conditioner and reconstructive conditioner. Day-to-day styling calls for a dime-sized bit of cream hairdressing massaged into the hair for moisture and shine. Trim hair every six to eight weeks to keep damaged, split ends at bay and to keep the shape of the hair as well.

Opposite: The elegance of the vintage pageboy. *Above right:* Healthy relaxed hair gives us many styling options.

ALL ABOUT WEAVES

More and more women are opting for weaves. They offer an easy way to add fullness and length to hair or to allow hair to grow out without worrying about or fussing with touch ups or trying to figure out a series of hairstyles. It has emerged as the answer to many hair dilemmas. The weave, which actually refers to wefts of hair sewn or braided into the hair, is probably the least understood of our various hair options.

Weaves are applied by the following methods.

• BONDING Wefts of hair are glued to the shaft of your hair close to the root. Benefit: This procedure is quick and adds volume and length. Risk: It can cause skin irritation.

• BRAIDING Your hair is divided into small sections and braided an inch or more with extensions and sewn or wrapped with thread to secure them. Benefit: Braiding is a healthier applica- tion than the glue used in bonding and/or the stitches used in sewing. Risks: Tight braids can con- tribute to traction alopecia and the chemicals used to maintain braids can damage your nat- ural hair.

• SEWING Wefts of hair are sewn onto a row of your cornrowed hair. Although it's time- consuming (anywhere from three to eight hours), this is the most popular and preferred method. Benefit: Sewing causes less damage than bonding. Risks: Sewing adds stress to your natural hair, and you run the risk of dam- aging your hair when cutting out the stitches.

There are two types of hair to choose from: synthetic fiber or human. Remember, the better the quality of the hair, the more expensive it will be. Opt for human hair, which can be treated like your own. Also consider the kind of hairstyle you want. If you want a sleek, straight look, buy straight hair. Don't make the weave any more work than it has to be!

You and your hair- stylist should consider your hair texture before adding mounds of hair. Make the weave compa- rable to your own hair. If your hair is thin, the stress of a too heavy

Left: A cascade of curls. *Opposite:* A corkscrew bob.

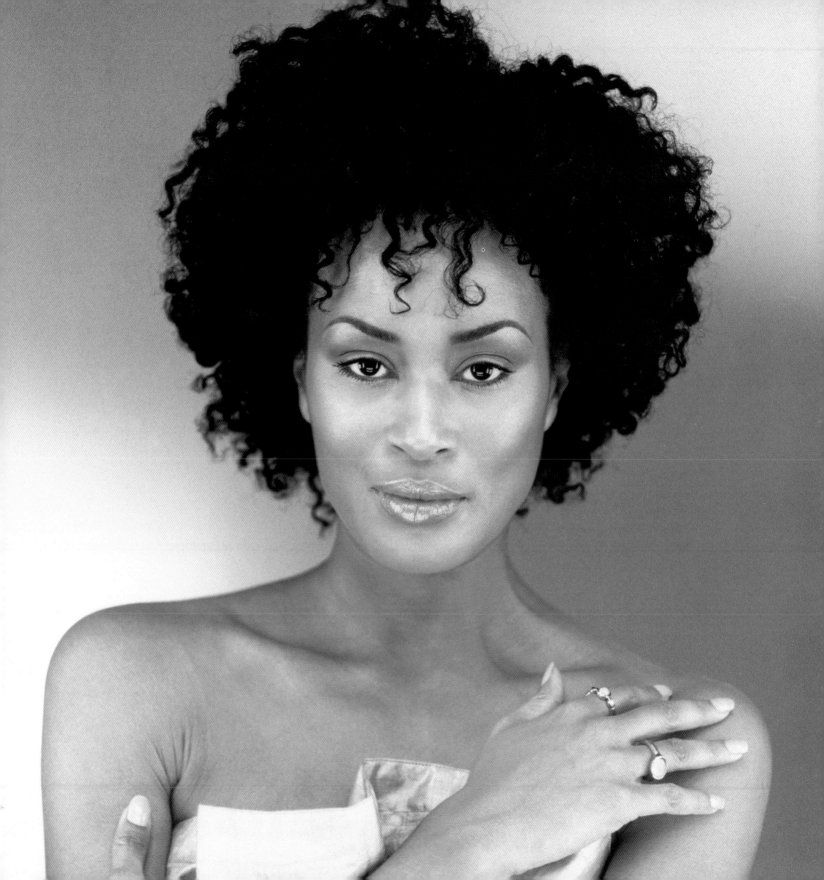

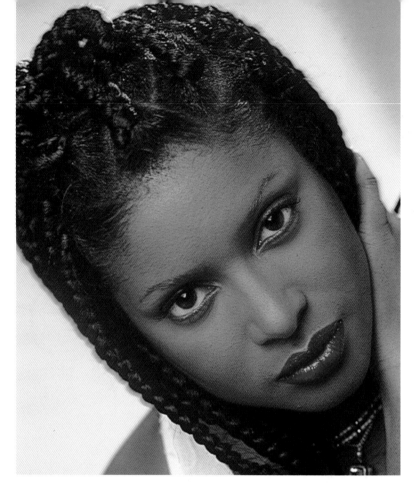

BACK TO OUR ROOTS
NATURAL HAIR AND BRAIDS

More and more sisters are opting out of their relaxers and falling madly and passionately in love with their natural hair. And they're having tons of fun with freedom Afros, sexy twists, and intricate braids that last for months.

CARE OF NATURAL HAIR Wash weekly for textured hair and at least every two weeks for braids and cornrows. To keep your natural hair soft and lustrous choose shampoos with extra

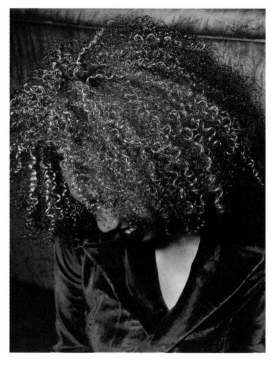

Above: Human hair braids. *Right:* Curly hair with golden highlights. *Opposite:* Locks in a bold and beautiful updo.

mane is going to pull on and weaken your natural strands. The most common mistake stylists make is adding too much hair. Find a stylist who specializes in weaves so that you get the best weave and care possible.

WEAVE CARE A weave should be washed and conditioned every week. Human hair weaves can withstand heat, styling gels, mousses, and lotions, but if you have a bonded or braided style, your natural hair is still exposed and it will be subject to damage. As your hair grows, the weave will loosen, so have it tightened in six to eight weeks. The recommended duration of a weave is four months.

emollients. Those formulated for dry or damaged hair are most nourishing. Pay special attention to the scalp. Follow with a wash-out conditioner. Once a month give yourself a hot-oil treatment. Moisturize hair daily with light natural oils like jojoba, sweet almond, palmachristi, or rosemary. For those wearing cornrows or individual braids, apply oil to the scalp and stroke braids in a downward motion until oil is gone. Keep styling gel on hand to smooth down frizzies at the hairline.

LOCK STEADY
HOW TO CARE FOR YOUR LOCKS

Locks command attention! Sisters with locks seem to just emanate confidence and a spiritual aura. That comes as no surprise, since locks are a symbol of the Rastafarians of Jamaica, West Indies, who consider their hair sacred. Nowadays, sisters all over the African diaspora are "unlocking" the power of locks.

The style gets its name in part from the process of strands intertwining permanently, locking, when combing, brushing, and other manipulations of the hair cease. Then every strand that would normally shed is caught up with the rest of the hair to form a strong, cordlike "lock." Once the hair begins to lock, the only way to change to a different style is to cut them off.

Your hair texture determines how quickly hair will lock. On average, it takes from four to six months, and the tighter the curl the quicker it will lock. Soft, wavy hair takes longer. You can begin the locking process by

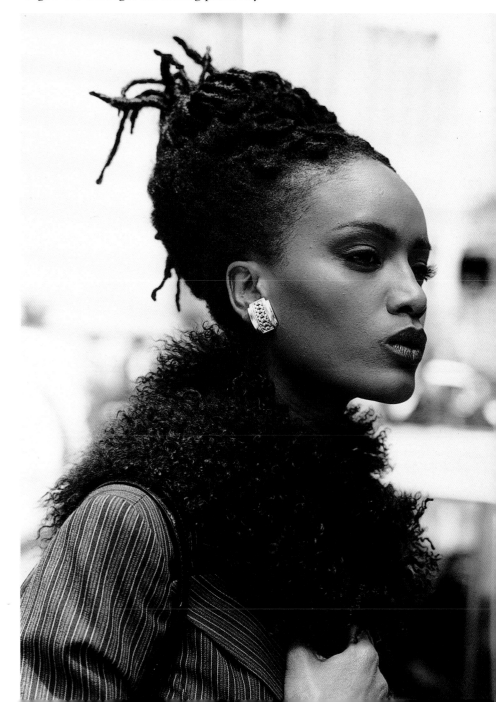

parting the hair and creating two strand twists or by palm rolling your sections of hair.

At the beginning of the process you must wait three to four weeks before shampooing the hair. In the meantime, clean scalp with an astringent and cotton swabs.

CARE OF LOCKS Cleanse hair with a shampoo for dry hair. Massage scalp gently to avoid breaking up lock sections. Towel-dry hair and apply a hot-oil treatment or a leave-in conditioner. Once locks have reached maturity (generally around the two-year mark), you can wash your hair as often as you choose and retwist as needed.

HAIR 911

Alopecia

Alopecia is a general medical term for hair loss of any type. Thinning hair, female-pattern baldness, and sudden hair loss are all forms of alopecia. Only a dermatologist can assess the type and the cause. A myriad of conditions can result in alopecia, so a complete medical history is required. Iron deficiency anemia, thyroid diseases, lupus, chemotherapy, and even crash dieting could be culprits. There are various types of alopecia.

ALOPECIA AREATA is thought to be an immune system disorder that causes bald spots to occur on the scalp. It is believed that the immune system goes haywire, triggering overactive white blood cells to attack the hair follicles. Rarely does total baldness occur, and hair usually grows back spontaneously. Alopecia areata may be treated by injecting cortisone shots until regrowth appears. For unknown reasons, certain medications that irritate the scalp may also cause hair regrowth.

ANDROGENIC ALOPECIA is male-pattern baldness that occurs around menopause. It is recognized as a general thinning of the hair, particularly in the crown and around the hairline. You'll never go completely bald, but your hair may get very thin.

TRAUMATIC ALOPECIA, or follicular degeneration syndrome, is the hair loss that quite frankly we inflict on ourselves based on the styling methods we choose. Years of repeated relaxing and/or coloring followed by heat results in chronic inflammation of the scalp. Hair loss is permanent if scar tissue replaces the hair follicle. The dermatologist may need to perform a scalp biopsy to determine if this has happened to you.

TRACTION ALOPECIA occurs when hair is pulled back too tightly—in slick ponytails, tight braids, weaves, and rollers. Bald spots are usually seen along the front and sides of the scalp. The hair is literally pulled out of the follicle, taking the bulb with it.

Alopecia areata, traumatic alopecia, and traction alopecia all require you to abandon damaging methods of styling. Give your hair a break from relaxers, color, or very tight braids. If your doctor has determined that scarring has not occurred, the hair will grow back. If it can't, ask your stylist for a new "do"—one that is healthier and camouflages any bald spots.

The drug minoxidil has been shown to help restore hair to those suffering from male-pattern baldness. Applied topically, the medication may stop hair loss and eventually new hair may grow back. But don't get too excited; while minoxidil works better for women than men, chances are you won't experience the regrowth of a mane reminiscent of your hair's glory days. Also, be prepared to take minoxidil for the rest of your life. Once you stop taking it, all of the new growth will fall out. Finasteride, an oral medication, has shown some promise in balding men; however, pregnant women should consult their physician because it may lead to birth defects.

Dandruff

What exactly is dandruff? Dandruff is dead skin cells that cause itching and flaking of the scalp. Dry scalp dandruff is characterized by white scattered scales that can be seen in the hair and on the shoulders. Oily scalp dandruff is recognized by large grayish-yellow oily scales that usually clump together in the hair. Basic over-the-counter dandruff shampoos that contain zinc pyrithione, tar, or salicylic acid are quick fixes. If you feel that dandruff is your constant companion, you may be suffering from seborrheic dermatitis, an inflammation of the scalp caused by regrowth of a yeast that normally lives in the top layers of the scalp.

Seborrheic dermatitis is generally character-ized by an itchy scalp and flaking in the scalp, eyebrows, and along the sides of the nose, ears, and mouth. There may be a mild redness of the skin. This condition is best diagnosed and treated by your dermatologist, who will prescribe a medicated shampoo and possibly a steroid cream to be used on the scalp to stop inflammation. If not controlled, seborrhic dermatitis can also contribute to hair loss, due to the damage of the follicles.

Breakage

Due to the inherent delicate nature of our hair and the various styling techniques we've adopted, a bit of breakage is not uncommon. While a split end here and there won't kill your look or your hair, it needs to be addressed and corrected immediately, before it becomes a problem.

SPLIT ENDS refers to strands that are split vertically in half. They are the result of overusing styling tools, scorching heat appliances, or vigorous brushing and combing. It's easy to combat them with a trim. If split ends are not nipped in the bud, they will run up the hairshaft, and eventually you'll lose the whole strand instead of a half an inch.

HAIR BREAKAGE is also the result of any of the above culprits and/or overprocessing, which leaves the hair dry and brittle. Again, the key is to condition once a week, alternating between protein for strength and moisture for pliability. Get regular cuts to remove the damaged hair.

LISA NICOLE CARSON

I TRIED TO RELAX MY HAIR ONCE, BUT THE CHEMICALS TOOK IT OUT. I GET IT TRIMMED EVERY TWO MONTHS AND KEEP IT MOISTURIZED. I RETURNED TO GREASING MY SCALP, AND MY HAIR WAS LIKE, "GIRL, WHERE YOU BEEN?" I COULD FEEL IT EXHALE. SOMETIMES YOU HAVE TO STICK TO THE TRIED-AND-TRUE.

HOW TO FIND A STYLIST YOU LOVE

A partnership with a hairstylist that you trust is key to achieving and maintaining healthy hair. Increase your chances of finding the stylist of your dreams by becoming an educated consumer. Go for the whole deal: a great cut and styling, a good level of comfort with the stylist and the price, overall professionalism, and a commitment to keeping your hair healthy. Don't sacrifice any of these elements; they are all necessary to make your visit to the hair salon a pampering experience and your relationship with your stylist a long and fruitful one.

One caveat: The best time to look for a stylist is when you're not desperate for one. For example, don't launch your search when you are in dire need of a touch-up, because that will supercede everything else. Nine out of ten times you will cave in to the first person you talk to, or overlook a serious recommendation (such as needing two weeks of deep conditioning before the touch-up) simply because you want your hair done now!

Here are a few tips to aid you in your search for a great stylist.

ASK AROUND Ask anybody—friend, family, or stranger—whose hair you admire for the name of her salon and the stylist there.

INTERVIEW POTENTIAL STYLISTS Once you find a few prospects, schedule get-to-know-you consultations. This will give the stylist an opportunity to examine your hair, ask questions about what you want and your hair-care history, and tell you what can be done to help you achieve your hair goals. The consultation gives you the opportunity to assess the stylist's personality, his or her specialties, the products recommended, and if the stylist's method of hair care is in sync with what you want. For example, if you like roller sets and the stylist is recommending blow-drying as the preferred method, then this isn't the stylist for you.

Also while you're chatting, take a good look around the salon. Note the level of professionalism of both the stylist and the salon overall. Remember, the stylist can be great, but if the shop gets on your nerves because they tend to overbook, or the staff is rude, loud, and gossipy, no matter how great your hair may look you won't feel good about your experience.

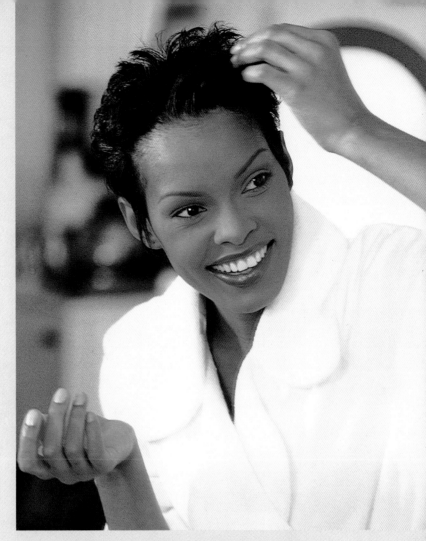

BE REALISTIC Once you have told the stylist what you want, be prepared to hear what the stylist can and can't do for your hair. Healthy hair should be your first and foremost goal. If the stylist is telling you that your hair is damaged and inches have to go, or you can't get your hair dyed and relaxed during the same visit, respect her expert advice.

BE PREPARED TO TELL YOUR HAIR'S LIFE STORY If you know that a regular-strength relaxer makes your fine hair limp, say so. Be up front about your hair mishaps, whether or not you take medication, as well as your likes and dislikes when it comes to hair care.

BE COURTEOUS Be on time. If you are going to be late or miss an appointment, call.

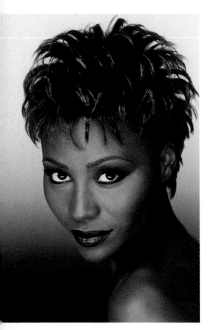

Above: A soft feathered cut with a hint of bronze highlights.
Right: Honeyed hues.
Opposite: Stunning salt and pepper.

COLOR FORMS

Today, more than ever, sisters are coloring their hair and loving it! With technology on our side, color has become the quick route to spicing up our looks. New formulas have been developed with an emphasis on conditioning benefits, rendering coloring products that are more gentle to our hair. And sisters have pulled out the stops. We're going platinum and golden and copper and every shade of bronze and brown we choose. Hair is no longer political. It's only about what feels good and looks good to you. To be sure, this is exciting, great news, but remember that hair coloring is still a chemical and that there are risks involved, so always consult a professional.

The safest color looks are subtle ones. Look for hair color that is one to two shades lighter or darker than your natural color for the safest, most natural-looking results. If you opt to color your own hair, consult the chart on the back of the product box. Below are a few things to consider for optimum results.

• Go a shade lighter than your actual hair color to add brightness and highlight grays in a lighter tone within the shade.

• Go a shade darker than your actual hair color to add richness and depth.

• Conditioning is key. Alternate weekly between strengthening and moisturizing conditioners.

Blonding is a tricky process, especially for those of us with dark relaxed hair. Why? The stylist has to use a lightener like hydrogen peroxide, to lift the natural color out of the hair. In order to get to a lighter shade, the hair must go through several levels (shades). Black hair is level 1 and it goes through brown, red, red-gold, until level 7, the palest yellow. Once the hair reaches level 6 or 7, the color is applied. Because of the amount of work and care necessary, the best candidates for blond are those with light brown, golden hair, and sisters with short natural hair.

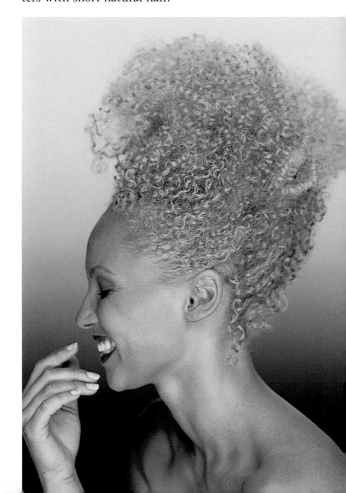

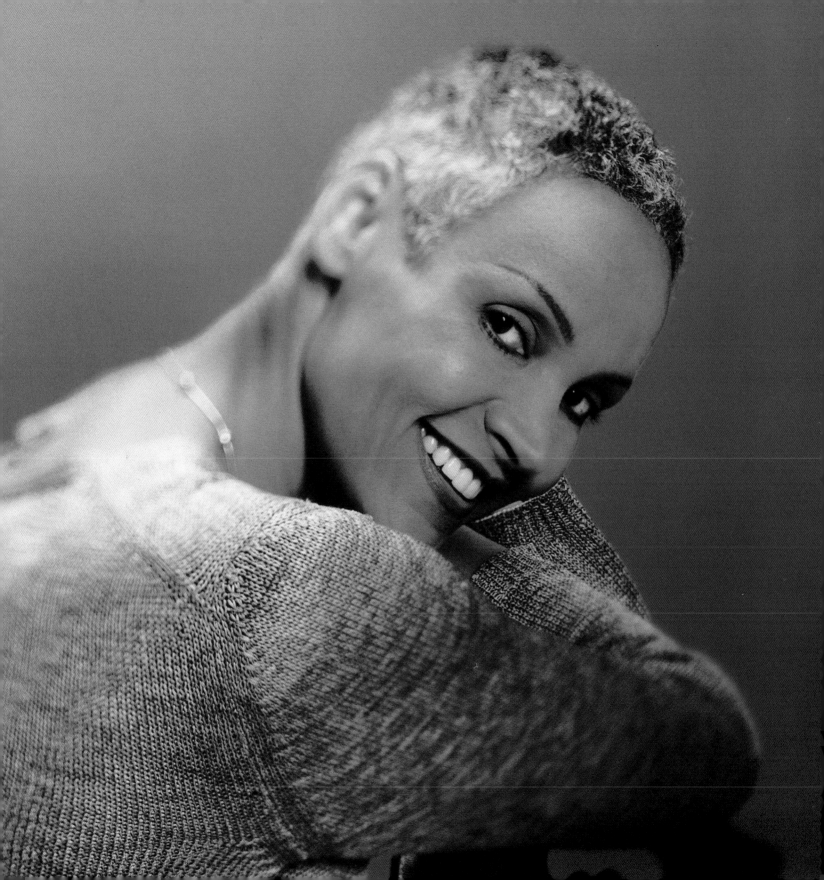

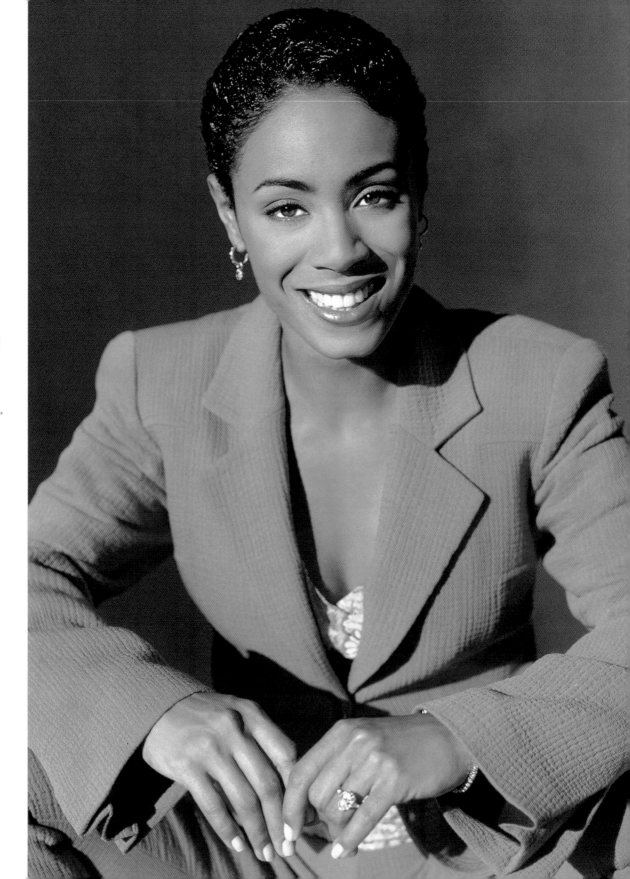

JADA PINKETT SMITH I'VE BEEN EVERY HAIR COLOR UNDER THE RAINBOW, BECAUSE I LIKE TO KEEP IT FRESH AND EXCITING. I KEEP MY HAIR SHORT SO I DON'T HAVE TO USE CURLING IRONS; I JUST GET UP AND GO.

HAIR COLORING

Color Type	Cautions	Results	Maintenance
SEMI-PERMANENT	• Virtually no damage done to hair	• Deposits color • Enriches natural color • Improves shine • Lasts six to twelve shampoos	• Use color-enhancing shampoos to keep color from fading
DEMI-PERMANENT	• May contain 5 to 10 percent peroxide • Do not apply for at least two weeks after a relaxer • Do not apply to hair previously colored with metallic dye	• Delivers longer-lasting gray coverage • Adds luster • Lasts through more than twenty-four shampoos	• Refresh color with a semi-permanent in the same color family • Condition hair weekly with a strengthening conditioner
PERMANENT	• Wait two weeks if hair has just been relaxed • Do not apply to hair previously colored with henna	• Penetrates the hair shaft • Lightens and/or significantly darkens hair • Covers gray hair • Requires touch-up every four to six weeks	• Condition hair daily with a spritz of leave-in conditioner • Follow-up with an intensive conditioner weekly to fortify hair with protein

EXPERT ADVICE

"You can take a dip in the pool without damaging your hair. Slick hair down with a creamy conditioner to act as a barrier between the chlorine and your hair, cover it with a chamois cloth, and then put on your swim cap. Once you have finished your swim, rinse your hair using a moisturizing shampoo, and follow with a conditioner." —Barry Fletcher, hairstylist, Avant Garde Hair Gallery, Capitol Heights, Maryland

"How do you know your hair is overprocessed? Breakage. Hair that can't maintain curls and has frizzy ends is overprocessed. The remedy is simple. Condition, cut, condition!" —George Buckner, hairstylist, Hair Fashions East, New York

"Hair needs a bit of oil on the scalp, especially when you exercise or if you perspire a lot. It will protect the hair from the drying salt in perspiration." —Olive Benson, hairstylist, Olive's Hair Salon, Boston

Opposite: Jada Pinkett Smith, actress.

"Sisters are moving from relaxing to pressing the hair, thinking that the hot comb is less damaging. Not necessarily so. Pressing the hair with the hot comb is still damaging because of the high degree of heat used. And we have a tendency to go for the hot comb or curling iron touch-ups between shampoos, which is not good. Limit exposure to heat because it can cause permanent hair loss." —Dr. Denise Buntin, dermatologist, Nashville

"Hair grows from the scalp, and breaks off from the ends. You can stop hair-end breakage by cutting the ends every four to six weeks and conditioning the shaft. A good trim will stop your ends from splitting." —John Atchison, hairstylist, John Atchison Salons, New York and Los Angeles

"I don't use petroleum, mineral oil, or lanolin. They are too greasy, too heavy, and they clog the hair follicles. Instead, in my products I use extra-virgin olive oil and castor oil mixed with fine herbs like jaborandi, maidenhair fern, sage, and nettle to stimulate hair growth, walnut leaves to strengthen the hair, and rosemary to make it luxurious." —Crystal Devin, Crystal's Royal Secrets, New York

THE MAKEOVERS

From Paris, France, to Paris, Texas, sisters are celebrated for their exquisite, exceptional hairstyles. But even though we make it look easy, we know that having great hair is a labor of love. *Essence* sent five sisters to stylists to get expert advice on how to tame their manes.

Stephanie

Stephanie had been keeping a natural for two or three years. But lately her hair seemed to have a mind of its own and she felt the need for a dramatic change. When she met with Ellin LaVar of LaVar Hair Designs in New York City, Ellin explained to her that many times natural hair has ends that curl back on themselves, so that when you're picking out an Afro, tension is created in the hair—and that means breakage. Together, Stephanie and Ellin decided on something totally new: a full-hair weave with smooth, natural textures.

First, Ellin washed Stephanie's hair with a moisturizing shampoo and conditioner. After drying, Ellin's assistant worked an oil-based moisturizer into Stephanie's hair to soften it and make it more manageable, then blew the hair out and straightened it with a hot comb.

With Stephanie's hair clean and soft, Ellin braided her hair into small horizontal cornrows,

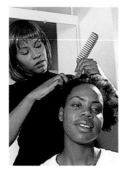

Above: Before. *Below:* Ellin LaVar styled Stephanie with a casually sophisticated weave.

and then sewed in shoulder-length sections of natural human hair. After the weave was successfully layered, Ellin blew it out then brushed it before giving the hair shape with a scissor trim.

To maintain her new hairdo, Stephanie washed, pressed, and blew out her new hair every two weeks—although she could have washed it more frequently. She also wrapped her hair each night to keep its flair and finesse.

Stephanie was amazed by the elegance and cool sophistication she felt with her new style, and even though she said she wasn't a "hair person," she had to admit the results were, well, unbeweavable!

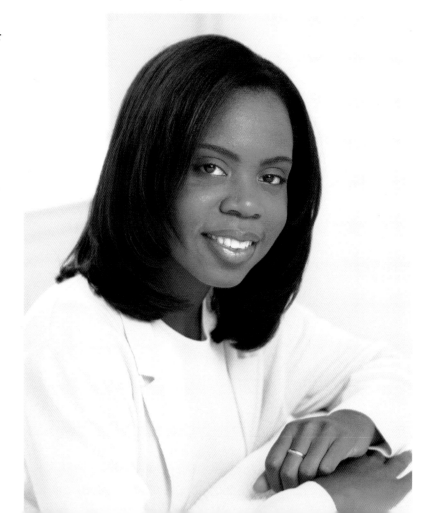

Victoria

Braided extensions are a common way many sisters maintain a fabulous style without the fuss. Braids can be tricky though, because synthetic extensions don't "breathe" the way real hair does. If they aren't groomed or treated properly, you can face excessive dryness and breakage around the hairline (known as traction alopecia). Victoria had long, thick, heavy extensions with new hair growth underneath in some places, and balding in others. With practiced care, Diane Bailey of Tendrils House of Ujamma in Brooklyn, New York, revitalized Victoria's hair and had her looking positively diva!

Diane gave Victoria's hair a chance to rest from the tension in the braids by taking out all of Victoria's old extensions with a combination of water and oil (at home try almond or sesame), then washing the hair with a peppermint shampoo to stimulate the scalp and prevent flaking. Treating the hair with a shea butter moisturizer and brushing the hairline with a soft toothbrush helped bring moisture all the way to the scalp's edges. Next, Diane used a deep protein conditioner for hair strength followed by a thirty-minute all-natural cherry mango hot-oil treatment to keep the scalp lubricated. A light rinse left some of the treatment in, and Victoria was ready for her new look.

Diane used naturally kinky human hair for Victoria's new look. To accent her statuesque beauty and give volume to Victoria's face,

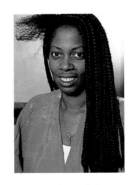

Above: Before. *Below:* Diane Bailey created a carefree finger style for Victoria.

Diane focused less on length and more on layers of twists to frame her face. And because her own hair was integrated into the extensions, it regained health while hiding the damage from the earlier braids.

Diane called this a "finger style" because its maintenance is so simple Victoria didn't even have to use a comb, just her fingers to keep the twists together. Diane also suggested Victoria use a light oil or hair butter for sheen, and a water spritzer for added moisture. With another wash, condition, and retwisting session after two months, Diane said Victoria's new look could last for up to four months of fuss-free fashion!

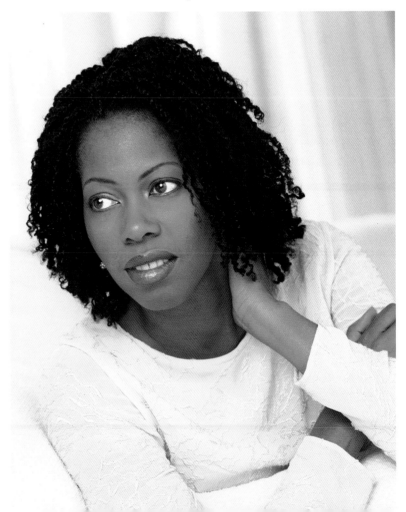

LaShena

LaShena had a soul sister's Afro. But natural hair needs moisture as much as relaxed hair does, and LaShena's hair was dry and brittle. The hair's color had grown out halfway, she had split ends, and there was a breakage problem caused by pulling her hair back with a headband or into a fabric headwrap. This led to a thinning and uneven hairline, especially around the front of her head. Diane Bailey of Tendrils House of Ujamma in Brooklyn, New York, came to the rescue and turned LaShena's hair don't into a hair*do*.

Diane immediately saw that LaShena's hair needed strengthening, so after a cleansing shampoo she gave her a protein treatment containing bone marrow to build the hair back up. She alternated the protein with a hot-oil moisturizing process during the next visit, so after four visits over two months LaShena's hair was healthy enough to be colored with a medium golden brown to wash out the brassy red and orange tones.

LaShena's hair was ready for Diane's African curl. Diane blew the hair out to loosen the curl, then she did a double strand twist and used gel at the ends of each twist to define the tips. LaShena's hair was thinner on one side, so Diane pulled the twists apart to give the hair body on that side while giving the fuller side an offbeat, funky style with microbraid cornrows from the front to an upsweep in the back.

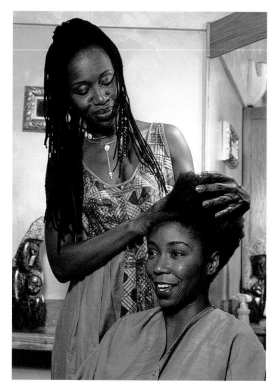

Above: Before. *Opposite:* Diane Bailey gave LaShena a funky, offbeat style.

This kind of combination gave LaShena the option of wearing the double twists for a couple of weeks, and then pulling the twists apart to create a different look and lengthen the life of the hairdo.

The maintenance for this style was easy. LaShena didn't have to use a comb or a pick— she just had to keep her twists even and together. Imagine, a hairdo that only needs fingers to keep it up! With a little gusto and a pinch of panache, Diane gave LaShena hair that accented her natural beauty and made a statement for keeping in touch with her roots.

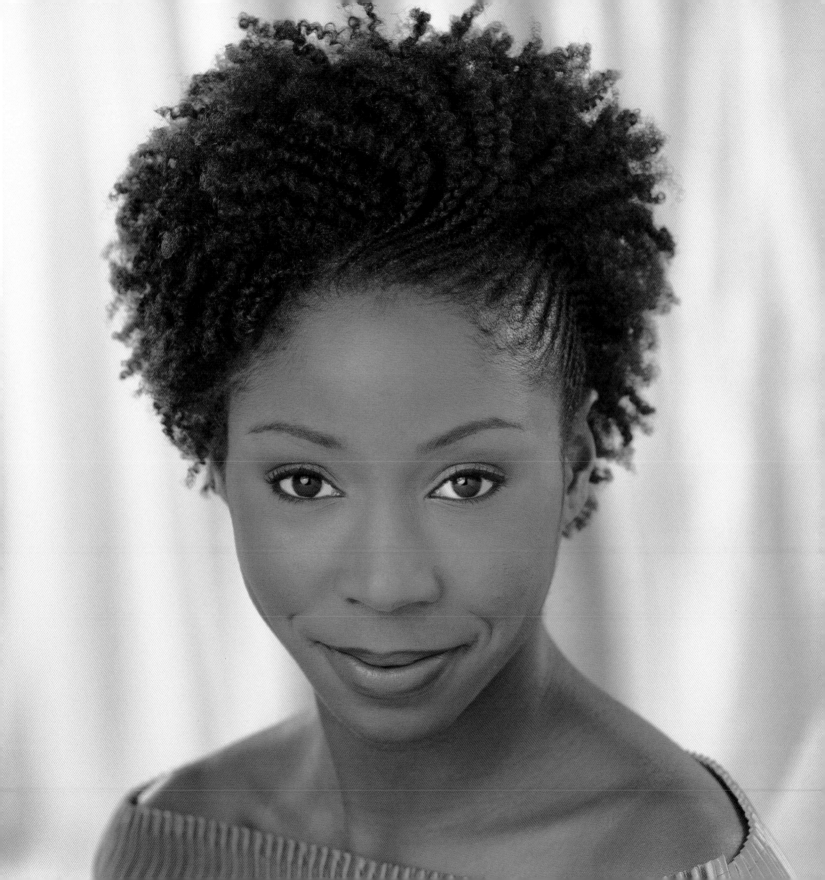

Natasha

Natasha's hair was in transition. She was working toward a natural by growing out a texturizer. Even though she wore her hair in twists or plaits, clipping her own ends left her hair uneven and without shape or form. And because Natasha's hair had been over-processed, it suffered from excessive dryness and breakage. Diane Dacosta of Dyaspora Day Spa in New York City rejuvenated Natasha's natural in a fresh, contemporary look that matched her sassy attitude.

Diane saw Natasha every three weeks for three months. She began restoring the much needed moisture to Natasha's hair with a conditioner cocktail made from herbal protein and the essential oils of flowers and other plant parts. To lock in that extra wetness, Diane had Natasha sit under a steamer for thirty minutes, where the intensity of the vaporized water penetrated deep into the hair shaft. After the hair became more manageable to work with, Diane evened it out by cutting off the two inches of texturized hair still remaining.

Natasha wanted her new-growth natural in a hassle-free style she hadn't tried before. Diane achieved this with tight coils lying close to the head and cascading from a part over her left eye. Maintenance was easy: Natasha wrapped her hair nightly to keep the coils sculpted. She also used a little emollient each day for added sheen and an organic mois-

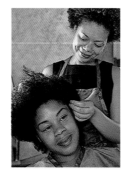

turizer to keep her scalp healthy and happy.

The results were phenomenal. Diane had taken Natasha from the no-woman's-land between a relaxed hairdo and an Afro and restyled her to lend a natural elegance to her bubbly personality.

Left: Before. *Below:* Natasha sports fabulous coils, thanks to stylist Diane Dacosta.

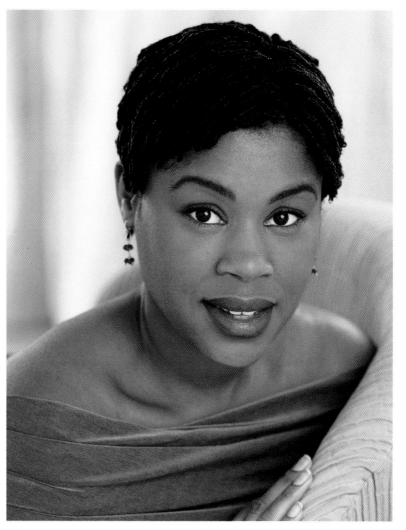

Belinda

Belinda wanted a radiant and exciting new look. She had been trying a lot of things to get a look she was happy with—a relaxer, a peroxide bleach job, gel for sculpting—but everything combined only dried out her hair, causing breakage and leaving toxins on her scalp. George Buckner of Hair Fashions East knew what she needed to get back on track to beautiful hair.

George began with an aromatherapy session to revitalize Belinda's scalp. He told Belinda that using the essential oils of herbs and fruits like chamomile, thyme, peppermint, and bitter orange opened the blood vessels and delivered needed nutrients to cells in the skin. This was followed by a lymphatic massage in which he rubbed the glands in the neck, forehead, and back of the head in a rhythmic, downward motion to increase blood flow and stimulate toxin-fighting hormone production in the scalp.

To strengthen the hair itself, George gave Belinda three sessions of an oil base and a reconstructive treatment with vitamin K. This process repaired the hair while moisturizing the scalp, which alleviated the itching and soreness Belinda suffered from the chemicals she had been using. After four sessions, her hair was healthier and strong enough for George to put in a mild relaxer.

With Belinda's hair straight and strong, George was able to cut it for style. This took

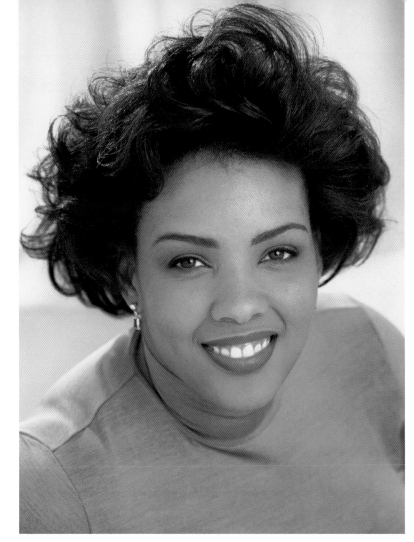

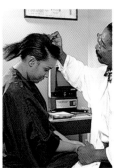

Above: Before. *Top:* George Buckner gave Belinda an exciting new look.

another four sessions, because he cut out the damaged hair and split ends gradually so that the change was not too dramatic. Belinda had her work cut out for her, too: She shampooed and conditioned her healthy new-growth hair at home more often, and she stopped using gel and other damaging products. The mild relaxer George gave her was enough to leave her hair manageable and fun to work with, and she made the most of it with a soft, unstoppable style.

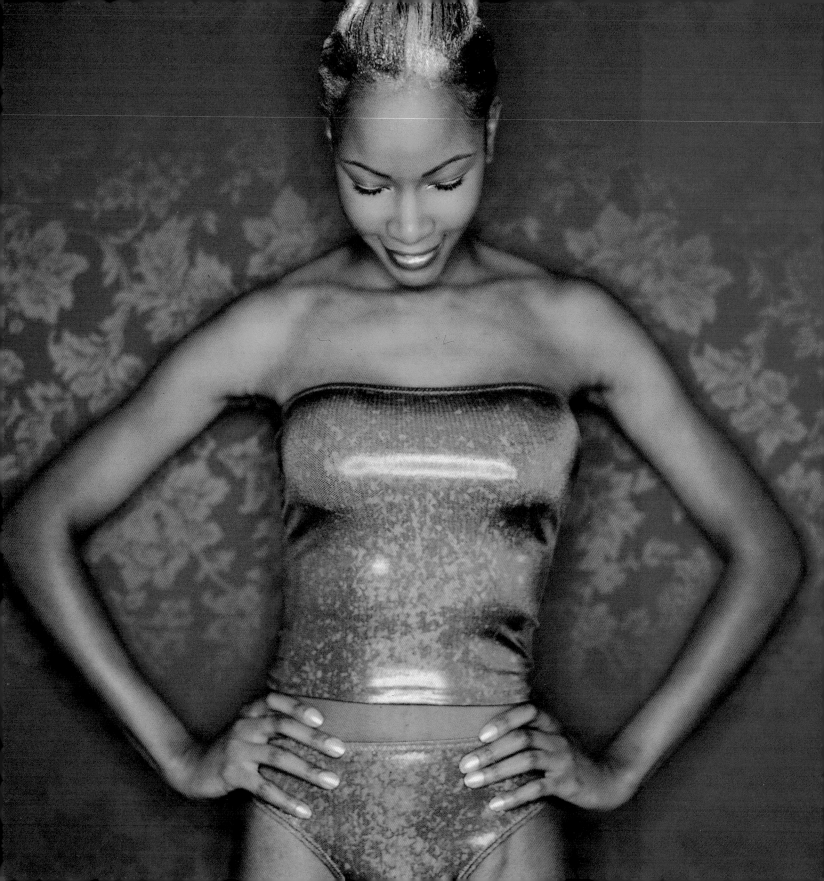

3 BODY BEAUTIFUL

LOOK IN THE MIRROR. There it is—your body. It's an incredible machine capable of doing amazing things: running a marathon, remodeling a house, bearing children. Your body is there to support you as you chase your dreams and pursue happiness. Yet the bottom line is you have to take care of yourself. Family and friends may love you a lot, but no one can take care of you as well as you can.

Just as you honor your God, so you must respect God's temple, the bodily place where your spirit rests. Exercise, good posture, preventative health, and pampering nurture your body while replenishing your soul and mind, and it all supports the growth of a vibrant, empowered woman.

SELF-ASSESSMENT

Do you feel healthy?

Do you feel good about your body?

Do you have good posture?

Do you sit up straight, with your feet planted on the floor at work?

Are your computer, keyboard, and chair set up in a way to avoid reaching or slouching?

Can you walk up a flight of stairs or break into a light jog without shortness of breath?

Do you exercise at least three times a week for a minimum of twenty to thirty minutes?

If time, health, or finances are a concern in starting a new exercise program or joining a gym, have you considered the benefits of walking?

Do you stretch well enough, watch your form, and wear supportive shoes in order to avoid sports injuries?

Have you pampered yourself recently? Do you do something nice for yourself a long bath, a manicure or pedicure, even a trip to the spa at least once a month?

Have you consulted a specialist about your varicose veins or other bodily concerns that refuse to respond to diet and exercise?

If you can answer yes to at least five of these questions, you have a good head start in your quest for a healthy body. If most of your answers were no, read this chapter as your first step toward attaining a new level of strength and fitness.

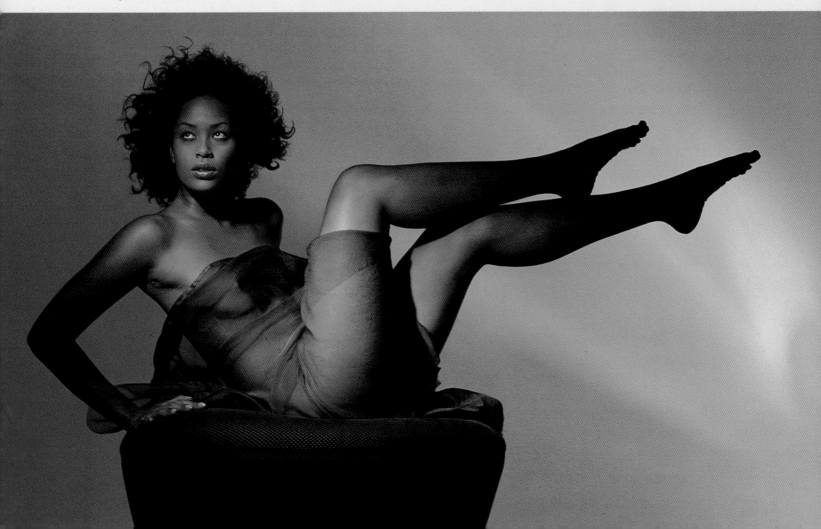

Medical doctors, naturopaths, and personal trainers may have very different ideas when it comes to what it takes to have a firm and fit body, but each would agree that an active body needs an active mind. A positive attitude about yourself fuels the energy and enthusiasm you'll need to make the changes you want and need in your life.

It's also important to recognize just how interconnected the body and mind are. Many times excess weight gain is not solely the result of unhealthy eating patterns and poor exercise habits, but also of a high-stress lifestyle that leads to overeating. Dealing with life's challenges in a healthy way is a prerequisite to getting the better health and fitter frame you're looking for.

POSTURE PERFECT

Carriage is as important as curves, and poor posture is like putting an evening gown on a broken hanger. Standing erect has a natural slimming effect, helping your weight drape more evenly and attractively. There's also the added impact of the grace and confidence you present to others. Lastly, poor posture can have an adverse effect on respiration, digestion, circulation, and can even lead to injury.

If you suspect your posture needs some work, start by thinking about how you sit and stand. Your shoulders should be open and back, and in a straight line over your pelvis. Concentrate on tightening your abdominal muscles by imagining that you are trying to make your stomach and the small of your back meet. Imagine yourself walking like a queen and you'll find yourself being treated like one!

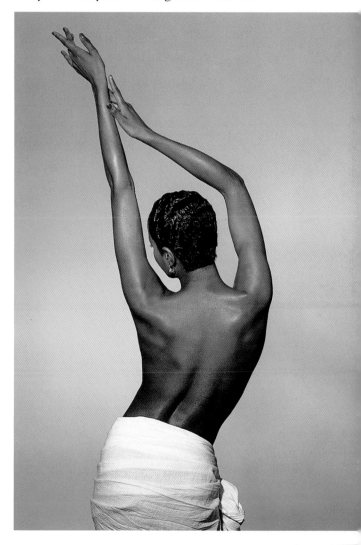

EXERCISE: A NEW BEGINNING

Here's how to get started on a new-you attitude. To get a good idea of the proportion of muscle and fat in your body in relation to your height and weight, calculate your body mass index (BMI). BMI = your weight in pounds $\times$ 703/your height in inches, squared. BMI is a good fitness indicator; a BMI of 22 is ideal, while a person with a 25 is about 10 percent over their ideal body weight. Someone with a BMI of 27 or higher is at least 20 percent over their ideal weight and considered obese. Blood pressure should be at least $^{120}/_{80}$ or lower, cholesterol under 200, and blood sugar under 110.

As you get started with healthier eating and integrating exercise into your daily schedule, remember it is more desirable to be a fit size

Below left: Awaken to a new sense of wellness. *Opposite:* Walking tall makes you feel graceful and confident.

fourteen or sixteen than an unhealthy size four or six. Your first goal should be to feel better and have more energy. As you awake to a new sense of wellness, from there you can begin to enjoy a greater feeling of physical fitness.

Physical activity can be divided into two types. Aerobic exercise builds your heart and lung power through moderate sustained activity such as walking, jogging, swimming, and biking. Anaerobic exercise is considered to promote muscle growth and definition and is characterized by the short bursts of intensity found in low repetition weight lifting, pushups, and crunches. The best exercise programs combine both types of activity for all-around holistic fitness.

To begin a new exercise program, aim for twenty minutes to half an hour of exercise three times a week. After you reach a comfortable plateau, shoot for sixty minutes four to five times a week. Remember, frequency is as important as intensity; in other words, ten minutes a day is a better effort than half an hour of exercise per week. Start small if you need to, with a ten-minute walk each day after lunch or dinner. Over time add on the minutes until you've reached a solid thirty minutes or more. You'll notice that you feel better and see slight changes within weeks of starting a new program, but for an even more visible difference, be patient and allow yourself at least six to twelve weeks depending on genetics and your fitness level. Moreover, think of your

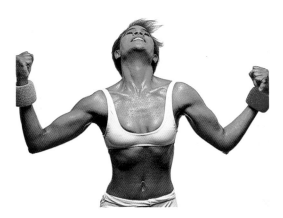

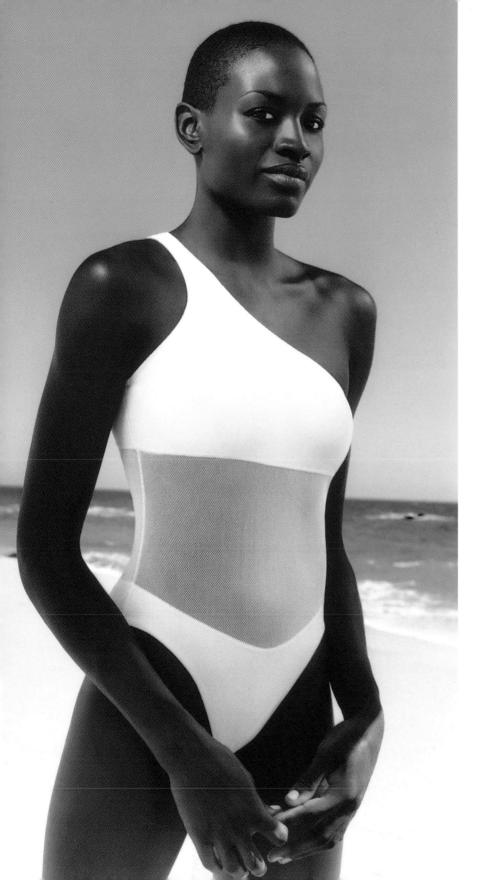

progress not just in terms of pounds shed. Are you more flexible? Do the muscles in your arms and legs feel stronger? Can you exercise longer without getting winded?

Before you start any program, don't forget to check in with your doctor. She will ensure that your heart and lungs are okay, as well as help you decide which exercises are best for you. She will also give you encouragement and helpful hints based on your medical history. For example, a person taking potassium supplements should have plain water after a workout, not drinks with the extra potassium many popular sports drinks contain.

As you begin your personal fitness odyssey, always remember to warm up adequately before jumping into your workout routine. A warmup might be a brisk walk, a light jog, or a quick spin on a stationary bike—anything to get the blood flow going and prepare the body for the workout to come. The warmup only needs to be about ten to fifteen minutes long; when you break into a light sweat, you're probably ready to begin stretching.

After you've completed your warm up, you'll want to give your body a good stretch before your workout begins. Stretching properly both before and after exercise (or any time at all!) will not only feel good, but it will also improve your flexibility while decreasing your chance of injury.

There are many exercises you can start at home as part of your fitness program. Body weight exercises that focus on specific muscle groups—

STRETCH IT!

Here are some stretches to try. Move into each position gradually and hold it for twenty to thirty seconds without "bouncing." Repeat each stretch at least two or three times.

LOWER BACK Lie on your back and bring your knees to your chest, wrapping your folded legs in your arms.

LOWER BACK AND REAR Lie on your back. With your right leg extended, lift your left leg and bring it across your body. Keep your shoulders on the ground and you'll feel the stretch in your lower back and buttocks. Switch legs and repeat.

HAMSTRINGS Sit upright and keep your right leg extended as you bend your left leg in until your left sole touches the inside of your right knee. Reach out for your right foot with your right hand and you'll feel the stretch in the back of your leg. Switch legs and repeat.

QUADRICEPS Stand up and hold on to a wall or a stationary object. Reach behind and grab your right ankle with your right hand, pulling gently as your thigh muscle stretches. Switch legs and repeat.

CALVES Place your right foot in front of your left as if you're taking a giant step. With your hands in front of you on a wall or some other stationary object, lean forward and feel the stretch spread through your left (back) calf. Remember to stretch each calf at least twice.

ARMS Bring your right arm across your chest and pull at your elbow with your left hand. Switch.

CHEST Stretch your arms out to your sides. With your hands on either side of a door frame, lean forward lightly and feel the pull in your chest and armpits.

---

push-ups, squats, and lunges—are easy to do and they'll help you tone, tighten, and add muscle definition. Here are some areas of the body and a few basic exercises to help you get moving.

Abdominals

Get rid of the sit-up. Most experts now think the old sit-up method was too harsh on the back and neck, and it didn't fully work the abdominal muscles. It's more effective to see your abs in three parts: upper, lower, and obliques.

LOWER ABDOMINALS This is the lower half of your stomach. Lie on your back with your knees bent. If you like, you can hold a fitness ball (found at any sporting goods store) between your thighs and calves to help your

form. Contract your lower stomach muscles, bringing your knees toward you. Do three sets of ten to twelve reps, working up until you can do twenty reps.

UPPER ABDOMINALS This is the part of your stomach that extends up to and under your rib cage, the place where your "washboard" is most visible. Lie on your back again. Simultaneously lift both your knees and head off the floor. You want to raise your head and shoulders to about a 45-degree angle, just enough to feel the squeeze yet without meeting the knees. Concentrate on contracting those upper ab muscles. Do three sets of ten to twelve reps, working up until you can do twenty reps.

OBLIQUES This works your sides, giving

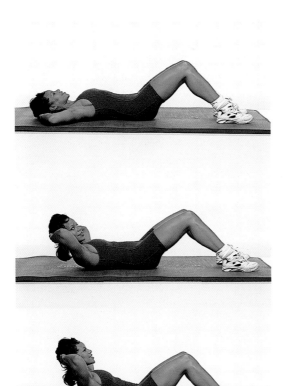

Left, top to bottom: Fitness diva Donna Richardson demonstrates the crunch. 1. Lie on your back with knees bent and heels on the floor. 2. Pull your abdomen in, and slowly lift your head, neck, and shoulders until your shoulder blades clear the floor. 3. Exhale as you lift, and inhale as you lower your body. Do eight to fifteen repetitions, rest briefly, and repeat. *Below right:* Exercise expert Kacy Duke demonstrates arm exercises with light weights.

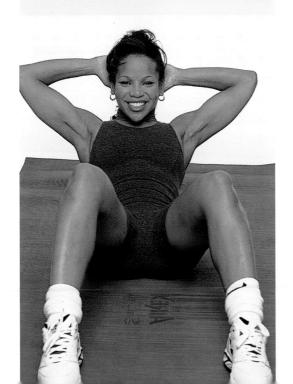

you more chiseled curves. Lie on your back with your knees bent. Put your arms behind your head. Raise and twist your left elbow toward your right knee. You should feel the squeeze in your left side. Do ten to twelve reps (again, building to twenty), then switch to the right elbow and left knee. Do three sets.

Arms and Shoulders

Inexpensive hand weights or even soda bottles filled with sand can be used to work the triceps, biceps, and shoulder muscles. Here's an exercise that works your biceps. Stand tall, with your back straight and your knees bent slightly. Hold a one- to three-pound weight in each hand, with your palms facing up. Slowly flex your elbows and raise the weights. Keeping your elbows at your sides, bring your forearm toward your shoulders, then slowly lower the weights to starting position. Repeat ten times and do three sets. Another great exercise for the chest and shoulders is the modified

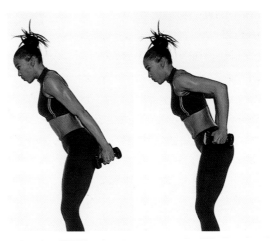

push-up. They're just like the push-ups you used to do in gym class, except you rest on your knees instead of on your feet. Keep your back in a straight line, and slowly lower your body to the ground on your arms before pushing yourself back up. Do as many as you can. Rest, and try to come back and do it twice more.

Buttocks

A favorite exercise of experts for tightening and raising the gluteal, or buttock, muscles are lunges. With your arms at your sides, take a giant step forward, keeping one foot planted firmly in place. As you bend your front knee, make sure that it doesn't extend past your toes. Squeeze your butt and use the squeeze to pull yourself back up. Repeat with the other leg. Do three sets of ten to fifteen repetitions apiece. (If you suffer from knee pain, do not try this exercise.)

Calves

Looking great in a pair of heels is easy. Hold on to a wall or a similar stationary object for support. While standing on a stair or other raised surface, rise up on the balls of your feet and

come back down again. Be sure not to rock back and forth—if you're feeling the stretch work through your calf, you're doing the right thing. Do three sets of ten to fifteen reps apiece.

Hips

The best strengthening and contouring exercise for your hips and thighs are squats. If you need to, hold on to to the back of a chair for balance, then, with your feet slightly apart and pointed outward, lower yourself toward the floor. Aim for a 90-degree angle but make sure your knees line up over your feet without going over the toe. Stand up slowly, holding your abdominals tight. Do three sets, ten to twelve repetitions per set. An added benefit: This one works the rear as well. (If you suffer from knee pain, this is not a good exercise for you.)

Thighs

Leg raises are wonderful toners. You'll want to do two varieties in order to adequately work and shape both the inner and outer thigh.

OUTER THIGH Lie on your side. Raise your top leg about eight inches. Do twenty slow

Below: Kacy Duke shows a great way to tone your abs, arms, and rear. 1. Sit on the floor with your arms behind you and your elbows and knees bent and your feet flat. 2. Inhale deeply, then push down with your hands and feet; lift and squeeze your buttocks while contracting your stomach. 3. Exhale as you slowly lower yourself. Unlock your elbows, and keep your abs and buttocks contracted until your bottom is on the floor. A complete movement up and down makes one repetition.

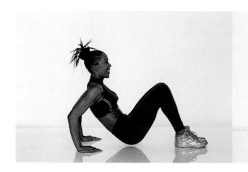 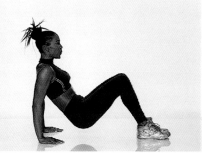 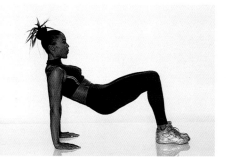

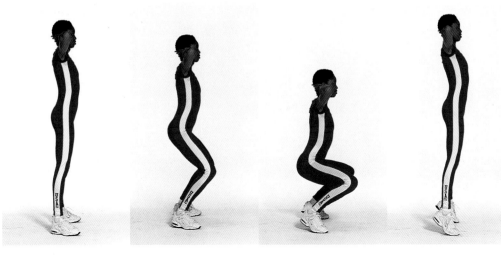

repetitions. Roll over and switch legs. Do three sets.

INNER THIGH Lie on your side, the top leg bent at the knee with knee on the floor. The bottom leg should be straight. Raise the bottom leg (you'll only be able to get it up four to six inches); feel the burn in the inner thigh. Do ten to fifteen reps and then switch legs. Do three sets.

For the aerobic part of your exercise routine, you may decide that you want a high-impact program or an activity that takes you outdoors. Think about your needs and desires when designing a program. You can choose heart-pounding, adrenaline-rush workouts, or you can have more gentle sessions. You might opt for a gym setting, but there is also plenty you can do outdoors or at home. The goal is to make working out convenient and a time you enjoy. Here are some of your cardiovascular workout options.

Above: Track and field star Kendra Mackey uses the squat to work the calves and back and front thigh muscles and to tighten the rear.
1. Stand erect with your feet a hip s width apart and your toes pointing outward. Clasp your hands behind your neck.
2. Slowly lower yourself while bending your knees. Keep your back straight, with feet firmly on the floor.
3. Bend knees as if sitting on a chair, until your thighs are as parallel to the floor as possible. 4. Raise your body, straighten your legs, and stand on your toes.

Walking

Walking might be called the perfect exercise. Gentle yet effective, it gradually burns the fat from your frame. Good for your heart and circulation, it's easy on the joints *and* on the pocketbook, and walking can be modified to fit the needs of pregnant, overweight, or senior sisters who may have special health concerns. Are you worried that walking is too easy and won't burn enough calories? Don't sweat it! A woman walking three times a week for an hour can take off a pound a week, and it's no secret that weight lost slowly over time is more likely to stay lost.

Running

Like walking, running is good medicine for the heart and circulation. It burns more calories than walking, and usually the weight loss is more rapid. Running, however, can be a strain on the body's joints, so try to run on packed dirt or level grass for a softer run; people with especially weak knees or ankles should avoid running on concrete. Use a treadmill indoors when the weather is cold or rainy. And don't try to do too much too soon; going for a marathon jog on your first day out is a surefire way to put yourself out of commission.

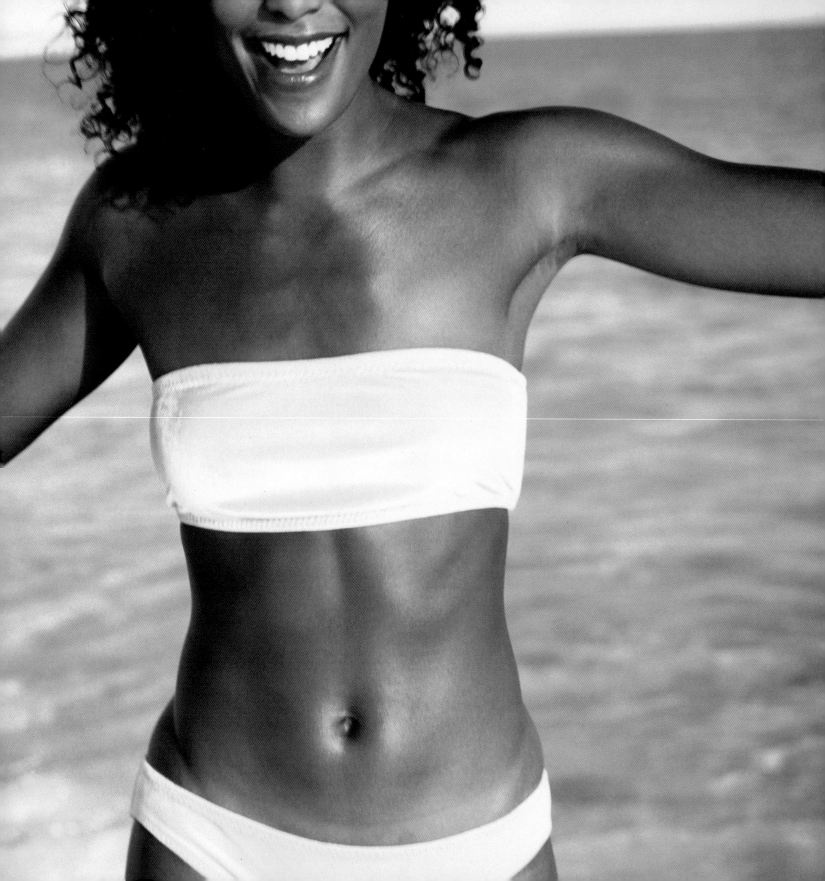

Step Machine

This machine is good for circulation and is intended to tone and tighten the calves, thighs, and rear. Head to the gym, select a program on a machine, put on your Walkman, and start climbing. Another option is a machine that allows greater program control and works the legs in a skiing motion. With either selection, remember that form is key. Ask a gym employee to show you the correct way to use the equipment. All cardiovascular machines are good for circulation. They help to make the heart and lungs work more efficiently.

Aerobics

This is a great workout that can be as low or high impact as you like. It's easy. Just find the right instructor or video where the intensity and complexity of the moves works for you. Many health clubs even offer varieties like gospel, funk, or hip-hop aerobics. Aqua aerobics are a great choice as well; the water adds resistance to help you burn calories and tone muscle, while at the same time it provides cushioning to reduce the physical stress and exhaustion you might get from other training activities.

Biking

Cycling burns a moderate number of calories and is a healthy way to exercise over the long

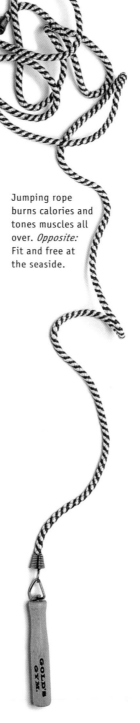

Jumping rope burns calories and tones muscles all over. *Opposite:* Fit and free at the seaside.

haul. It strengthens the legs well, gets the heart rate up gradually, and increases circulation and endurance over time. Outside, always ride wearing a helmet and obey local traffic laws.

Jumping Rope

Favored by boxers, this exercise is excellent for burning calories, getting your heart rate up, and pumping up your stamina. As an all-over toner, jumping rope works the arms, legs, and rear. Ropes are inexpensive and you can use them anywhere. Heavier, pregnant, or older sisters should be careful about jumping because, like many activities, it applies repeated pounding and stress on the back and joints. As always, the key is consulting with your physician or a trainer and using moderation, increasing your jump time as your endurance grows.

Boxing and Kickboxing

With lunges, jabs, and fancy footwork, boxing has become more popular for women as a workout technique. Kickboxing adds a self-defense, martial arts element as kicks and spins are brought into the mix. Sisters who work out this way report quite a drop in weight, not only from the amount of calories burned but also from the all-around fitness and body tone that the variety in training brings. For an Afrocentric twist, sign up for capoeira lessons and learn about the half kickboxing, half dancing martial art brought to Brazil by Africans hundreds of years ago.

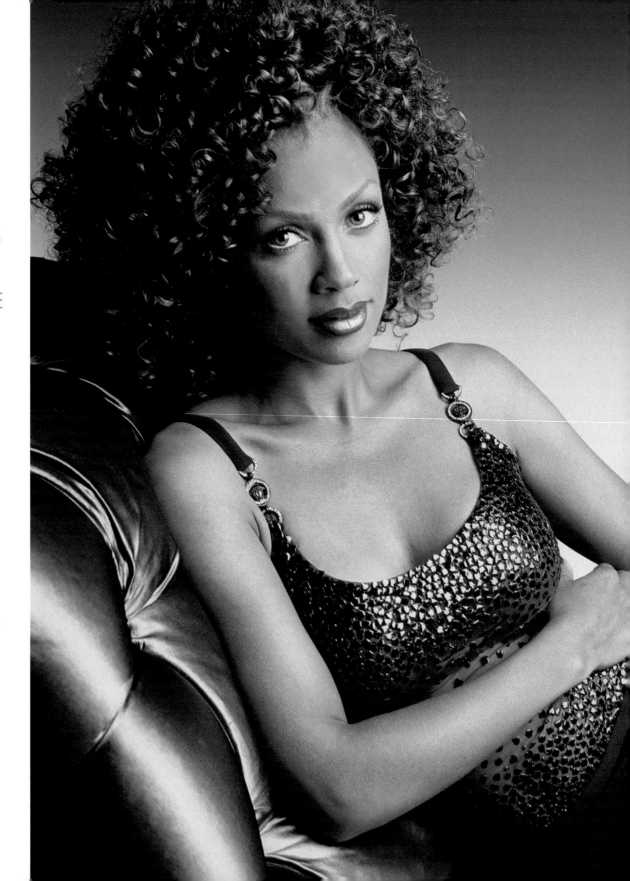

VANESSA L. WILLIAMS

I DO PILATES, AN EXERCISE REGIMEN THAT LENGTHENS AND STRENGTHENS MUSCLES THROUGH SLOW, INTENSE MOVEMENTS ON SPRING-RESISTANT APPARATUS.

Here are some other options to explore when developing your workout routine.

Yoga

An ancient meditative practice combining deep breathing and stretching, yoga is well known for its soothing effect on the mind. It's also terrific exercise for muscle strength, toning, and posture. As you become more comfortable and skilled in the positions, you may want to try power yoga, a more intense and athletic variety that will work your heart as well as any other cardiovascular activity.

Pilates

Developed at the turn of the century and previously used by dancers and athletes in physical therapy, Pilates (puh-LAH-tees) uses specially made machines and floor exercises to strengthen the stomach area and the buttocks while stretching the legs and arms. It provides strength, tone, and better posture through breath control, arm and leg extension, and working the deepest layer of the muscle. Once a well-kept secret, the low stress and no sweat aspects of the workout allows diehard devotees at centers around the country to quickly slip back to work or home feeling energized and relaxed after a session.

Weight Training

If you join a gym, you'll find a variety of weight-lifting options that provide targeted exercises for almost every part of the body. There are generally two types of weights: free weights (such as barbells, dumbbells, and bench weights) and weight machines (where the weights are part of the machine itself). A weight-training program can be designed to add definition and tone to your physique, or it can be used to increase muscle mass. For definition and lean lines without that bulky look, stick to the light weights and a high number of reps. Be sure to read the instructions carefully and ask the gym staff to help you the first few times you use the machines. It might even

Below: Lunging with light weights is a great way to tone hips and thighs. *Opposite:* Vanessa L. Williams.

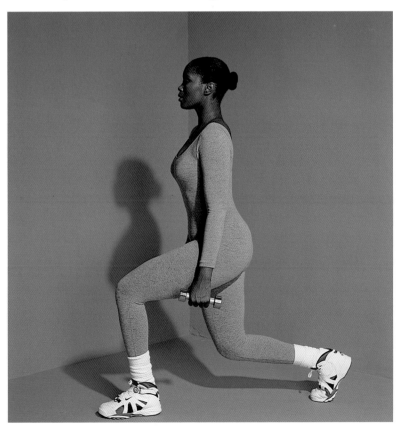

YOGA

Yoga, popularly considered to be an Indian practice of mental, spiritual, and physical cultivation, also has roots in ancient Egyptian (Kemetic) culture. Grandmaster Asar Ha-Pi, an expert of Egyptian yoga and philosophy at A New Horizon Health Institute in Chicago, teaches Egyptian yoga as a quiet, restful way to focus on improving the body and mind.

The mummy pose is a good one to get started with; it was used by ancient Egyptians as a way to retreat from daily stress. Begin by lying on your back on the floor. A mat or towel underneath you might make you more comfy. Separate your legs so that your feet are two to three feet apart. (If you have back problems, place a pillow underneath each knee.) Cross your left hand over your right with your thumbs touching. Slowly roll your head from side to side a few times to loosen the tension in your neck, then bring your head back to center. Relax your shoulders. Imagine your breath sweeping away the aches and pains from any tight areas in your body. As this energy circulates in your body, allow all your thoughts to float away as soon as they enter your mind. Lie quietly for a while, basking in this state of complete relaxation.

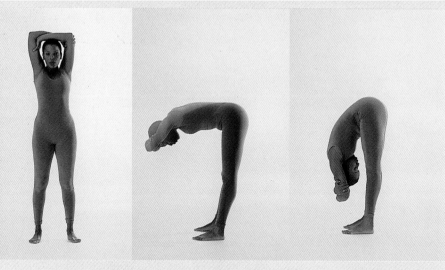

Try the forward pyramid bend to strengthen hamstrings and stimulate digestion: 1. Stand with your feet a hip's width apart and raise your arms above your head. Clasp your elbows with your hands. 2. Inhale, exhale, and slowly roll down from the hips, lowering your elbows as close to the floor as possible. 3. Keep your knees straight and feel your thighs muscles pull upward. Hold for at least fifteen breaths, longer if you can. Exhale and slowly roll up.

be worthwhile to pay a trainer to show you proper form for your first few sessions of pumping iron. Too much weight or bad form will quickly lead to injury.

A Note About Personal Training

Depending on how serious you are about becoming a fitness fanatic, you might want to consider hiring a personal trainer. A trainer certified through accredited programs like ACE or ACSM will help you by demonstrating the correct way to warm up, stretch, perform specific exercises, and use particular equipment. Because good form is central to a fitness program, a poorly done leg raise or crunch is really a waste of time; that's why you can't underestimate how much working with a trainer will help you, if only for three or four sessions. The most important thing is to find a trainer with good communication skills and a knowledge of anatomy and physiology. They should help you to achieve your potential— without making it too easy or too hard on you.

If you're on a budget, remember that the best things in life are free—or close to it. For a walking or running program, you only need to invest your time. Rent exercise videos. Consider buying exercise equipment secondhand. Look into the YWCA, which may let you exchange volunteered services for use of the facilities. And yoga and dance studios often offer inexpensive onetime classes.

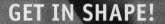

GET IN SHAPE!

Get a good start on your exercise program. Sharone Huey, a personal trainer in New York, stresses the importance of getting your heart and lungs in shape for the weight loss and body tone to come. Here are her suggestions for a six-week interval training program. Remember to include a warm-up/cool-down and stretching before and after the workout. Ready, set, *go!*

WEEK ONE: Alternate one minute of jogging with one minute of walking (this is known as active rest) for a total of twenty minutes. Pace yourself and aim to do this three to five times a week.

WEEK TWO: Cut down on the active rest. Alternate one minute of jogging with thirty seconds of walking for a total of twenty minutes. Three to five times a week.

WEEK THREE: Increase the workload. Jog for one and a half minutes; walk for thirty seconds. Twenty minutes, three to five times weekly.

WEEK FOUR: Repeat week three to allow your body to get used to the increased workload.

WEEK FIVE: Two minutes jogging, thirty seconds of active rest.

WEEK SIX: Repeat week five.

This program can and should be modified based on your results. Feel free to cut back or gradually increase the pace and duration of the workout depending on how your body feels. For example, you might build up to a five-minute run with one minute of rest, or your session can build to sixty minutes, up from the twenty you started at. As the intensity of your workouts increases, you ll notice changes in your body, such as deeper breathing and maybe even a little weight loss. You can also mix in the toning exercises described in the chapter after your workout, or during another time of the day.

THE POSTWORKOUT MUSCLE RELAXER BATH

Just because you re working out like an Olympian doesn t mean you won t feel a little ache in your muscles. Try the following bath at home with these essential oils.

2 drops rosemary
2 drops marjoram
2 drops lavender
2 drops chamomile
2 tablespoons canola, olive, or almond oil

Mix the oils and stir them into a warm bath. Soak and relax. For alternative combinations, try arnica, lavender, rosemary, juniper, and peppermint or lavender, chamomile, ginger, rosemary, almond, and St. John s wort oils. Either combination can also be used with a little extra vegetable oil as a massage oil.

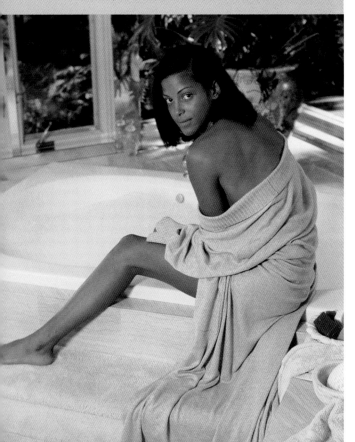

Left: A relaxing bath is a great way to unwind. *Opposite:* Basic body care is an investment in yourself.

BASIC BODY CARE

Congratulations! You're working your body, getting fit, and feeling stronger. But don't forget our bodies are delicate, so remember all the great care you've been giving yourself all along; everything from regular checkups with the doctor to setting aside special time for yourself is part of dignifying your temple and investing in your greatest asset—yourself.

Ears

Sisters keep our history alive with earrings, an ancient way of adorning the body. Most piercing specialists will advise you on how to keep the ears clean and infection-free while the hole heals. Be careful around young ones, as hoop earrings and the curiosity of small children are a bad combination. And remember some sisters are predisposed to keloids—dark, scarlike tissue that develops around the piercing. If you begin to form keloids, see a dermatologist, who will most likely treat it with topical steroids. For torn earlobes, a plastic surgeon should be able to repair the damage.

Elbows and Knees

Don't get caught off guard! These areas can become dry, flaky, and chapped, especially in cold weather. To go from ashy to classy, keep

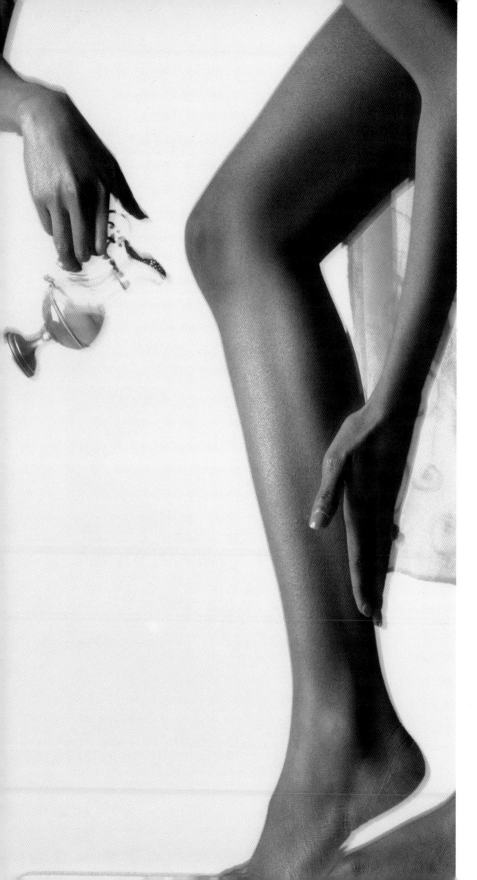

your elbows and knees soft with moisturizing lotions.

Eyes

Take care of the windows to your soul. Check-ups should be done yearly. If you need glasses or contacts, get them early to give your eyes the break they deserve. Nowadays the hardest part about imperfect vision is choosing from all the fashionable and lightweight frames available for the near- and farsighted.

Contacts come in hard and soft as well as daily wear, extended wear, and disposable varieties. Though some lenses can be left in for days, even a month at a time, many eye doctors advise removing and sterilizing the lenses nightly in order to avoid infection and keep your eyes healthy.

Lastly, talk to your ophthalmologist about the recent advances in laser eye surgery if you can't bear the thought of glasses or contacts. Radial keratotomy and photorefractive keratectomy are some of the newer sight correction procedures.

Feet

Our feet are the pedestal for the rest of our body weight and they take a great deal of abuse as we pound the pavement or exert ourselves in exercise. Try resting your feet during the workday and soaking them at night, especially if you're required to stand most of the day. Mix your high-heeled attitude with low-heeled pumps and flats when you can. Uncomfortable shoes may not only lead to painful walking, but foot problems like corns as well. Bunions are hereditary but are also affected by bad footwear. If you experience some discomfort, check for drugstore remedies like corn and bunion pads, creams, and ointments. If the problem persists or becomes painful, see a podiatrist.

Treat yourself to a pedicure every once in a while. Aestheticians use a variety of ways to beautify your feet, but watch out for salons using pumice stones and foot cutters. They're great for at-home pampering, but it's a smart health practice to keep your feet's business to yourself. And remember the simplest care: Keep your feet moisturized, covering them in lotion and putting on socks before bedtime.

Hands

In general you can keep your hands soft and sexy by using moisturizing lotion. In the harsh winter months, you might also want to consider special treatments like cream or paraffin wax manicures, which are meant to add and lock in extra moisture.

Nothing cares for the hands like a regular manicure. What's more, it's an elegant showcase for the finishing touches you're putting on your body. A well-done procedure should last at least a week. There is varying advice on how cuticles should be treated, but the general agreement is that they should be either

TONI BRAXTON
IT MAY SOUND CRAZY, BUT I USE SCOURING PADS—THE PLASTIC ONES, NOT THE WIRE ONES—ON MY FEET TO SCRUB OFF DEAD SKIN. AFTERWARD, I RUB MY FEET AND TOES WITH PETRO-LEUM JELLY, THEN SLEEP IN SOCKS.

lightly trimmed or gently pushed back—never severely cut or shoved back.

Nowadays there are a good number of inexpensive nail salons where manicures, pedicures, and waxing can be done for a fraction of the cost of upscale salons. What's the difference? Many times a higher awareness of cleanliness—new instruments for nail work, and disinfected work surfaces for each client—is found at the more expensive salons. A new nail file should be used each time, as well as the orange stick. Clippers, nippers, and instruments for pushing back the cuticle should be stored in disinfectant (the UV

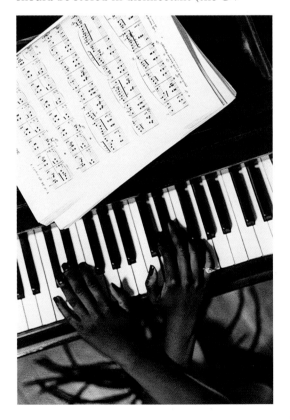

lights used by many salons are not proven to kill all germs). That's important: Repeated use of wax sticks and unsanitary conditions can transmit disease, and using instruments that haven't been adequately disinfected can spread infections as well. Don't forget to check sanitary conditions at the salon. A good salon will be happy to reassure that your health is their top priority.

Legs

For those who prefer smooth, shaved legs, as with your underarms, dermatologists recommend that you shave in the same direction as the hair grows. The result will be close to that of shaving against the hair, and you'll cut down on the risk of cuts or bruises, which can often lead to dark spots on African-Americans.

Skin

The body's largest organ, skin really communicates the state of your health to the rest of the world. With the positive changes happening in and around your life, you'll want to be sure to keep your sable skin radiant with the exuberance of the renewed you. See the chapter on skin for expert advice on daily cleansing, troubleshooting, and beauty tips.

Teeth

After your total body and spirit makeover, you'll probably be smiling a lot more. You know the routine: Brush and floss after every

JANET JACKSON
FOR ME, EXERCISE IS THE KEY, BUT THAT'S JUST HALF OF IT. THE OTHER HALF IS THE PROPER WAY OF EATING. I EAT FISH AND VEGETABLES WITH THE LEAST AMOUNT OF FAT POSSIBLE.

meal. Also, remember that your diet, beverages such as coffee and tea, and smoking all affect the brilliance of your pearly whites. Dental appointments should be scheduled every six months to keep cavities in check.

For a photogenic smile, there are many corrective options to think about. Whitening uses a bleaching solution to remove stains and discoloration from eating, drinking, and smoking. It may not be that effective to fix the darkening from a root canal or from the use of antibiotics during dental development. Either way, be sure to consult your dentist before using an at-home whitening kit.

Braces used to be kid stuff, but now it's commonplace for adults to use them to correct spacing, overbites, crooked teeth, or other problems. Your dentist can fill you in on braces with smaller, less obvious metal bits as well as lingual braces, which are placed behind the teeth. While the smaller braces can be as effective as the larger variety, there are some things to consider with the lingual type. They can sometimes cut and bruise the mouth and it can be harder to clean them, leading to food decay and halitosis. Ask your dentist about which will work best for you.

Lastly, if you have chipped, crooked, broken, or stained teeth, unsightly spaces or fillings, ask your dentist about crowns, veneers, implants, and bonding procedures. These modern-day miracles can have you smiling like a movie star at the next family reunion.

THE AT-HOME MANICURE

Why pay more? You can save money and might have more fun with your sisterfriends doing manicures at home. Here's a checklist and some tips.

> **cuticle pushers**
> **orange sticks**
> **cotton swabs**
> **cotton balls**
> **pumice stone**
> **emery board**
> **lemon slice (optional)**
> **oil (optional)**
> **cuticle cream**
> **hand cream**
> **nail polish**
> **base coat**
> **top coat**
> **nail polish remover**

• Remove existing nail polish and make sure all items are sanitized. Soak your fingers in a bowl of warm, soapy water. Add lemon to freshen and remove dark spots on nails. Soak dry, brittle nails in warm olive oil or almond oil. Dry hands and gently loosen any remaining dirt with an orange stick. Be careful not to prod into the nail bed.

• Select a thick cuticle cream. Massage it into each cuticle, moving the ball of the thumb in a firm, rotating motion to help circulation and encourage a healthy glow.

• File an orange stick to give it a smooth, rounded edge. Gently slide it slightly under the cuticles and push them back without forcing the cuticle too far. Do not use a cuticle remover, sharp stick, or metal instrument; that can open the nail bed to infection or chemical irritation. (Don't accept these methods from professional manicurists either.)

• Choose a hand cream for your skin type and rub in generously. Pull finger joints upward, then use the first and second fingers to push the skin down toward the knuckles, as if you were smoothing gloves onto your hands. Firmly massage the palm, using a rotating motion.

• Cleanse your hands to remove oil from the nails without stripping all the moisturizer from your hands. Apply a base coat to keep nails from absorbing pigment. Follow with the selected polish, allowing each coat to dry before applying the next. Finish with a top sealer; try a quick-drying one. Allow plenty of time for the polish to dry.

Experiment with color. Even if you need a plain, professional look, sample different approaches to "neutral" for your rich skin: clear, pinks, peaches, light beiges, mellow browns, classic reds, soft bronzes—perhaps gold for evening events.

THE AT-HOME PEDICURE

Treat your feet! Here's some advice on how to give yourself—or a friend—a well-deserved pedicure. Here's what you'll need.

> **1 bowl or foot tub**
> **Epsom or sea salts**
> **bubble bath (optional)**
> **baking soda (optional)**
> **cuticle pushers**
> **orange sticks**
> **cotton swabs**
> **cotton balls**
> **toe divider (optional)**
> **pumice stone or foot file**
> **toenail clippers or nail scissors**
> **rubber-tipped nail stick**
> **emery board**
> **cuticle cream**
> **witch hazel or rubbing alcohol (optional)**
> **hand cream or petroleum jelly**
> **nail polish**
> **base coat**
> **top coat**
> **nail polish remover**

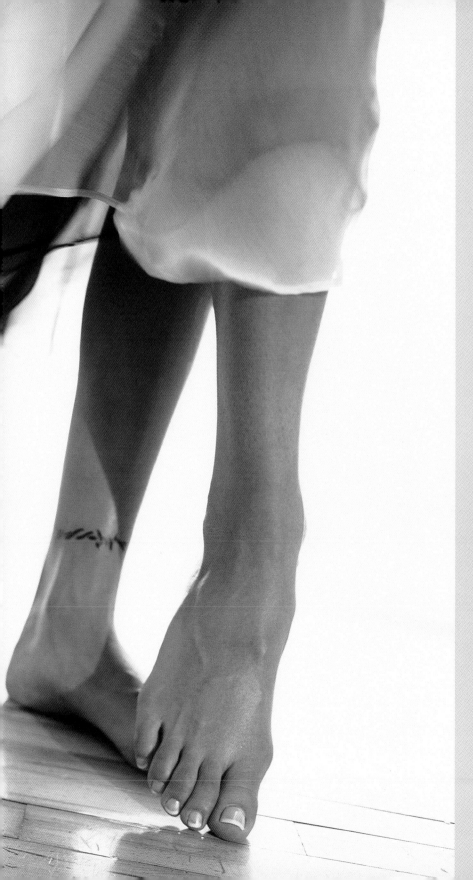

• Assemble and sanitize your equipment. You might even consider investing in a heated foot-massage bowl like professional pedicurists use. Remove any old polish from toenails.

• Prepare a traditional soak, using a cup of Epsom salts or sea salt to a gallon or 4.5 liters of comfortably warm water. Or, treat yourself to an aromatic soak, using about a half capful of scented bubble bath and two tablespoons baking soda to a gallon of warm water.

• Soak until the skin is soft, about twenty to thirty minutes. Use a pumice stone or foot file to remove hard, dry skin from the heels, sides of the feet, and the soles, avoiding the toes. (Do not use a razor or allow professional pedicurists to use one for this. Razors can leave cuts and introduce infections.)

• Carefully dry your skin, especially between the toes where fungi and bacteria flourish. Examine your feet for obvious problems like fungus, corns, calluses, or enlarged joints that may need professional care.

• Use a toenail clipper or nail scissors to cut nails square at the top, following the natural shape of the toe—no shorter than the edge of your toe. Avoid cutting back into the grooves of the toe, which can encourage ingrown toenails. Smooth the corners with a coarse emery board.

• Massage cuticles with cream, using a rubber-tipped nail stick if you prefer. Slide a smooth, rounded orange stick under the cuticles and push them back without forcing them too far. Do not use a cuticle remover, sharp orange stick, or metal instrument; that can open the nail bed to infection or chemical irritation. Rub the feet with hand cream or petroleum jelly, but avoid the space between the toes. If those crevices feel moist, try witch hazel or rubbing alcohol to discourage germs and fungus. Knead and massage the soles, heels, and insteps.

• Apply a base coat to keep nails from absorbing pigment. Follow with the polish, allowing each coat to dry. Seal with a topcoat or gloss. Allow plenty of time for the nails to dry, and moisturize your feet before putting on socks, hose, or shoes.

THE ROYAL TREATMENT

Pamper yourself! After all your hard work in the gym and out, you deserve an experience that can soothe and strengthen not only your strained and stressed body but also your mind and soul. Pampering is the icing on the cake to give you the peace of mind and renewed energy to be a better mother, wife, daughter, sister, coworker, and friend.

MASSAGE Many salons have a staff of massage therapists trained in making you feel like a natural woman. The Swedish technique involves gently rubbing the body, while Japanese Shiatsu uses deep pressure in specific points. Some massages combine a little of each method.

AROMATHERAPY uses subtle scents and fragrances thought to stimulate the brain and body to relieve a host of emotional and physical conditions, such as stress, depression, insomnia, and pain. Aromatherapy often incorporates essential oils to give a greater effect, such as sage for relaxation or rosemary for mental stimulation.

REFLEXOLOGY works on the belief that body areas and organs have corresponding pressure points in the feet, so a foot massage can target specific ailments such as stomach pain or headaches, as well as give you a greater sense of holistic well-being.

BODY TREATMENTS Soft skin and a healthy glow can be achieved with a number of body treatments. Using body scrubs, exfoliants like Dead Sea salt are mixed with oils and kneaded over the body to take away dead skin. Body wraps soften the skin by moisturizing the body and wrapping it in oil-soaked sheets and heated blankets. Another exquisitely exotic moisturizing technique is the mud bath, where the earth's own nutrients are used to enrich your skin.

WAXING Many salons offer waxing services for the underarms, legs, and bikini area. Waxing uses hot wax to catch and pull the hair out of the skin. Some sisters are starting to use lavender wax, where oil is put on the skin before waxing. The wax shrink-wraps around the hair and can be gently pulled off, while the skin is protected by the oil. A bit more expensive, the procedure is a good option for tender places like the bikini area and underarms. Rarer techniques are sugaring, the use of a natural honey wax, and threading, a Middle Eastern process using a thread to pluck the hairs.

In bikini waxing, there are a few styles you can select. Regular works well with fuller briefs or bathing suits. Narrow is a better option for women who prefer French or high-cut apparel, while Brazilian style leaves you with a thin strip of hair.

Opposite: Pamper yourself!

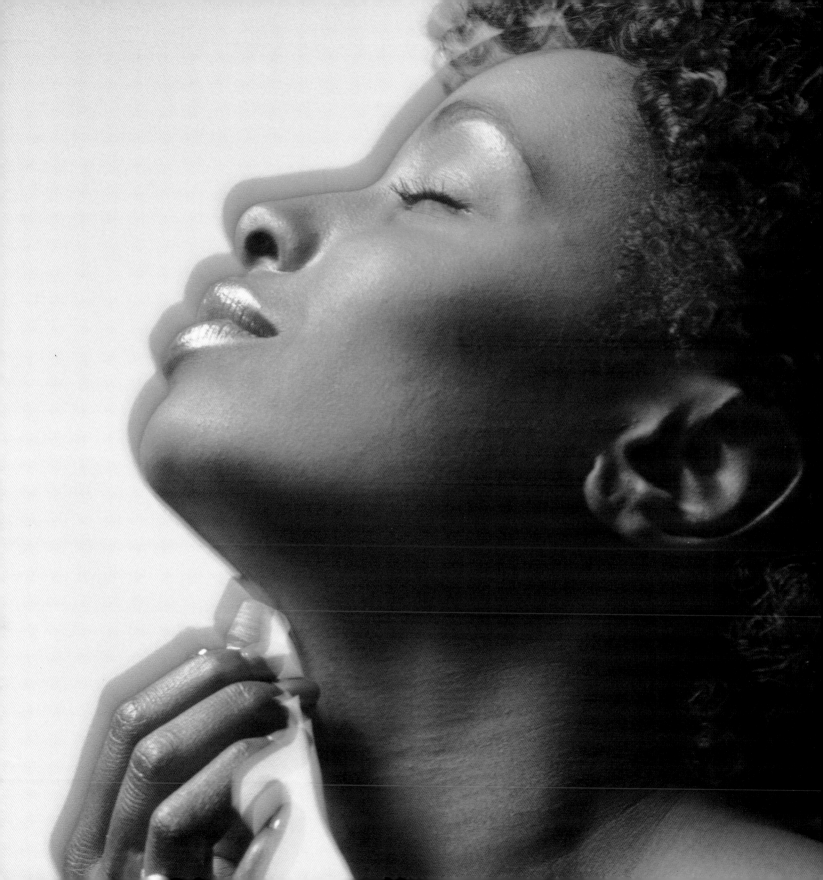

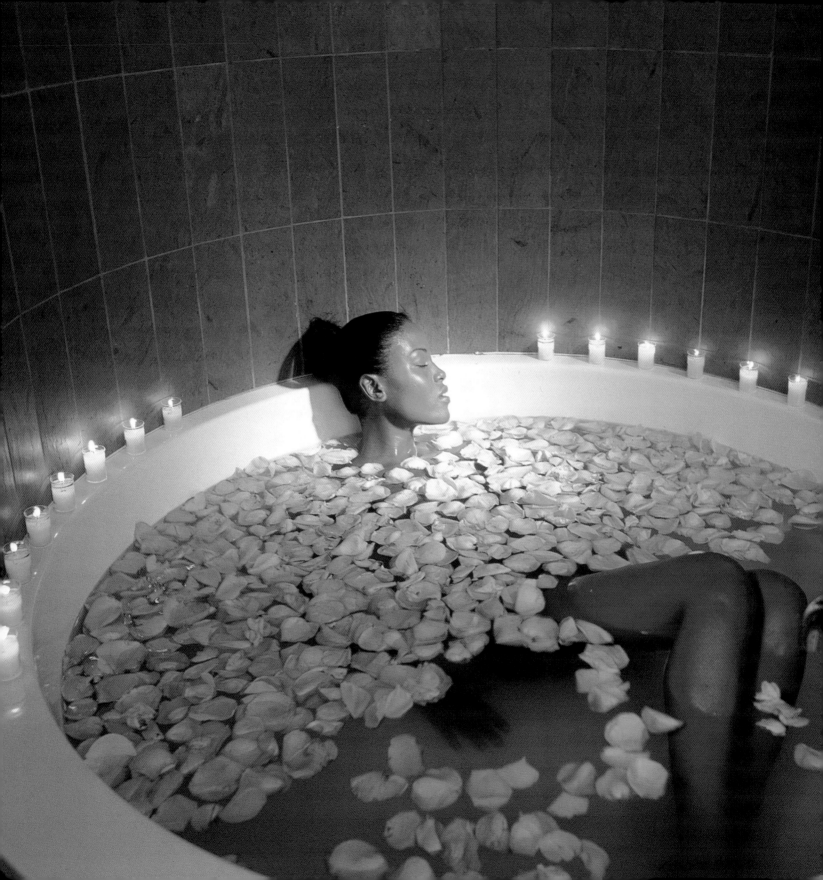

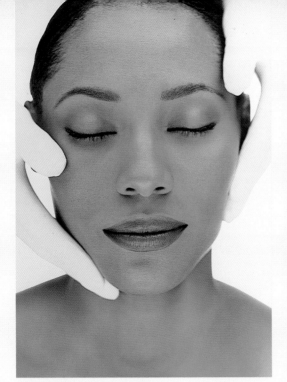

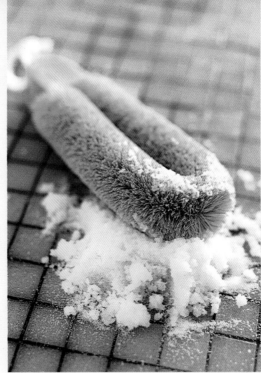

Opposite: Aromatherapy, combined with a warm bath, is a powerful stress reliever. *Right:* Massage can make you feel calm and relaxed. *Far right:* Exfoliants like sea salt wash away dead skin.

DO-IT-YOURSELF MASSAGE

Bonita Buchanan-Jones, a veteran massage therapist based in Michigan, offers a little trick to ease the vise that's squeezing your brain.

Using both hands, place your fingertips where your eyebrows begin just above your nose. Feel for the bone under the brow. Firmly apply pressure on that spot for a count of seven. Move your fingers a quarter of an inch along your brow bone. Again, hold for a count of seven. Move another quarter of an inch, again holding for a count of seven. Repeat until you've moved your fingers across the entire surface of your eyebrows. This technique is helpful if you feel a migraine coming on. Make contact with these pressure points several times a day until you feel relief.

Here's another easy acupressure practice if you're stressed out. With the thumb and index finger of one hand, grab the webbed area between your thumb and index finger on the other hand. Hold for a count of seven. Repeat the practice with the other hand.

DOWN-BY-THE-SEASIDE BASIC BATH SALTS

Salts have a long and distinguished history as an aid to relaxation and rejuvenation. Commercial bath salts can be expensive and limited in the scents offered. Try this for an easily customized and cost-effective alternative.

$\frac{1}{2}$ **cup Epsom salts**
2$\frac{1}{4}$ cups of sea salt or table salt
$\frac{1}{2}$ **cup powdered milk**
$\frac{1}{2}$ **teaspoon essential oil (lavender and/or rosemary are recommended)**

Mix ingredients and place them in a dark bottle that is clean and dry. Let the mixture stand a week to ten days. Use $\frac{1}{4}$ cup of the mixture in each bath. For aches and pains, add $\frac{1}{2}$ cup dried eucalyptus leaves and hops and $\frac{1}{8}$ cup each of garden sage, thyme, and lavender to one cup Epsom salts.

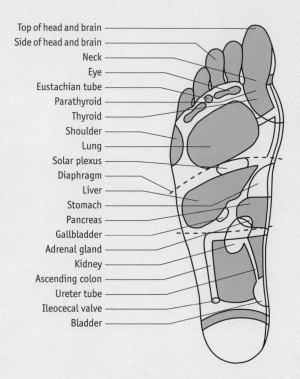

Top of head and brain
Side of head and brain
Neck
Eye
Eustachian tube
Parathyroid
Thyroid
Shoulder
Lung
Solar plexus
Diaphragm
Liver
Stomach
Pancreas
Gallbladder
Adrenal gland
Kidney
Ascending colon
Ureter tube
Ileocecal valve
Bladder

Pituitary gland
Sinus
Ear
Trachea
Bronchial tubes
Heart
Esophagus
Stomach
Pancreas
Spleen
Waist
Transverse colon
Descending colon
Small intestine
Sigmoid colon
Rectum
Sciatic nerve

WHAT IS REFLEXOLOGY?

The term *reflexology* is based on the theory that reflexes in one or both feet correspond to other parts of the body: heart, lung, pancreas, and so on. Various techniques using thumbs, fingers, and hands are used to apply pressure on the reflexes for a specific organ, gland, or other body part. Stimulating those nerve endings is intended to stimulate circulation and aid natural healing, as well as promote spiritual harmony. The techniques are best done by professionals, but if you would like to sample the technique at home enlist a friend or partner and try this: Gently massage the whole foot; apply pressure in the designated reflexology points, using the forefinger joint or the thumb. Allow about thirty minutes to complete both feet.

ESSENTIALLY YOURS OIL

To make your own essential oil, steep flower petals, citrus skins, or herbs in safflower or olive oil for at least a day. Strain and reserve the oil. Discard petals, skin, or herbs and replace with fresh ones every other day for at least ten days. When the scent is strong, discard the solid material, measure oil, and mix with an equal amount of ethanol. Cap tightly and shake once or twice daily for two weeks. Spoon off the alcohol or use an eyedropper to remove it. What remains is the essential oil. Most recipes use about ten drops of essential oils for every ounce of carrier oil like canola or olive oil. Equipment such as beakers and stoppers can be found in chemistry supply shops.

Right: Spas offer wonderful pleasures such as this water treatment.

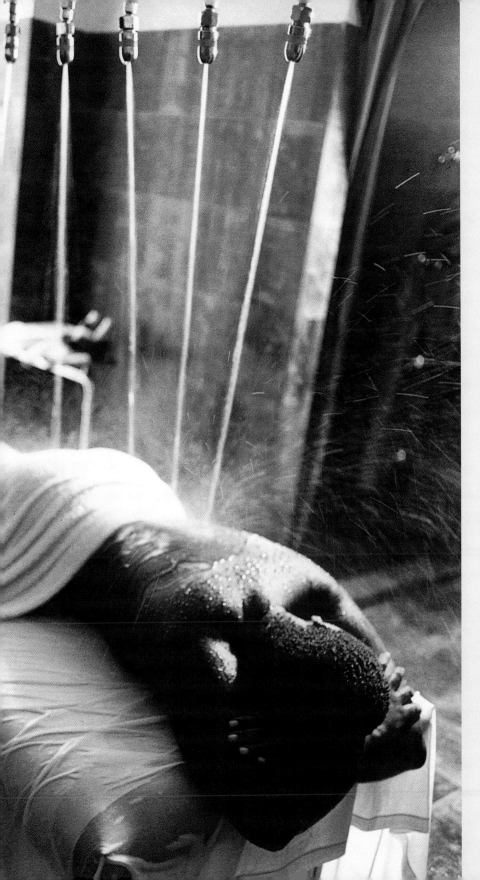

NEW BEAUTY BODY MASK

If a trip to a spa isn't in your budget, you can still enjoy some spa secrets in your home. Here's some ideas for a do-it-yourself body mask.

2 teaspoons honey
2 tablespoons yogurt
1 teaspoon vegetable oil
$\frac{1}{3}$ cup powdered clay (found at many health food and beauty stores)
$\frac{1}{2}$ cup mineral water or floral water (such as rose, lavender, or chamomile waters)
10 drops of essential oils

Mix honey, yogurt, and vegetable oil. Add clay slowly, alternating with small amounts of water to form a smooth, thick, creamy paste. Slowly add drops of the essential oils. For cold or flu relief, try eucalyptus, thyme, lemon, and rosemary. For an uplifting and energizing mix, use rosemary, bergamot, and lime. Mix well. Massage lightly into hands and arms, then feet and legs. Spend a minute or two on each body section. Work toward the heart and body center.

Leave the clay on and recline on a towel for fifteen minutes as you meditate or pray. You can spend the time in a warm tub of water, but some of the clay will wash off. After rest or the bath, rinse the clay off in a warm shower without using soap. Pat dry and wrap yourself up in a warm robe or blanket. Rest fifteen to thirty minutes more to get the full effect.

Finish with a body scrub. To make an exfoliating scrub, try $\frac{1}{4}$ cup sea salt, $\frac{1}{4}$ cup medium-ground cornmeal, $\frac{1}{3}$ cup olive oil, and 10 drops of essential oils. Standing in a tub or shower, apply with a gentle scrubbing motion, working from the extremities inward toward the heart.

Step out of the shower and into a new you!

BODY 911

Like any machine, the human body needs tune-ups and detailed care. Here are some common challenges that may keep your body from achieving its maximum potential.

Athletic Injury

Exercise and weight-loss programs can make you look good, feel great, and still be loads of fun. Pace yourself, and always be sure you're well stretched and using the equipment in the right way. If something hurts, let it rest and get it checked out by a doctor. Overexerting yourself and ignoring pain are sure routes to a sideline setback.

Cellulite

This is the dimpling often seen in the hips and buttocks. Diet and exercise are probably the best way to smooth out your legs, as beauty creams and liposuction are said to offer only temporary or minimal improvement. Doctors also cast a skeptical eye on methods using rollerlike objects to break up the fat, as well as on anticellulite massage. Some women report that their thighs look better after these procedures, so if you are open to alternatives see what a dermatologist or a spa near you has to offer.

Liposuction is best for women in their optimal weight range who have pockets of fat that diet and exercise just can't seem to remove. A solution is injected into the area to be treated, then fatty deposits are vacuumed out with a small needle through a tiny incision. At one time the procedure left scars and required a hospital stay, but now most of the small incisions tend to heal nicely and the operation can be done on an outpatient basis. As always, think about diet and exercise before going under the knife, because liposuction should not be used as a sole weight-loss technique.

Repetitive Stress Injury

This term covers a range of injuries in the body's soft tissue, like ligaments and tendons. RSI is caused by long-term, repeated physical exertion, as well as general wear and tear. Often associated with RSI is carpal tunnel syndrome, an injury that affects the hands and wrists in everyone from violinists to computer programmers. Tennis elbow, a painful outer elbow condition, is caused by overstress of the forearm muscles.

Signs of an RSI are tightness, trembling, muscle soreness, aching, tingling, sharp pain, and other such symptoms in the hands, arms, neck, and shoulders. If you suspect you have an RSI, see a doctor immediately; the care you receive early on can make the difference between a few days of discomfort and the need for surgery or long-term physical therapy.

Preexisting medical conditions like diabetes, arthritis, thyroid disease, gout, excess

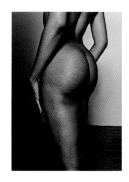

Your body is a finely tuned machine and a work of art as well.

weight or sudden weight gain, hormone conditions, and smoking may increase risk of injury. Job conditions such as stress, infrequent breaks, and fast and monotonous work are other risk factors.

Take preventative measures by looking into using an ergonomic workstation at the office. If you use a computer, make sure you don't have to arch your neck in order to see the screen—optimally it should be at eye level (with a glare resistant screen to reduce eye fatigue). Your chair should be designed to support your back as much as possible; the back cushion should be firm, shaped to align with your spine and reach to the middle of your shoulder blades. When typing, keep your arms parallel to the floor, shoulders and wrists relaxed, legs uncrossed, and your hips level with your knees. Invest in a phone headset and your neck will thank you. Above all, take a break every thirty minutes or so. Go get a glass of water or take a three-minute stretch. Lastly, if you're the kind of working woman who takes a good deal of work home at the end of the day, think about the weight distribution in your bags. Consider dividing it into two carryalls or even investing in a travel-size business suitcase (on wheels) to get your materials to and from the office.

Shin Splints

This common sports injury, resulting in lower leg pain, can be caused by inadequate stretching, intense exercise, or frequent change in terrain while running. They're easy to take care of: Just reduce the intensity of your workouts, stretch well, and ice your shins when you're finished. More serious are *stress fractures*—actual hairline bone breaks that come from high-stress activities like long-distance running or repetitive jumping exercises. Always make sure you have the proper shoes to absorb impact, and if the pain persists try to see a doctor before things get worse.

Varicose Veins

These veins, which can range from "spider" veins just under the skin's surface to knotty, more visible veins, can be reduced with sclerotherapy—injections of a saline-based solution that helps the veins constrict. This is a good method for sisters wary of laser therapy, which works with lasers to seek out the redness that's somewhat more visible in the skin of white women.

Weight Loss

A healthy diet of reduced calories as well as increased exercise has shown to be the best method for weight loss. Have patience! Shakes and crash diets may provide temporary slimming, but the weight often quickly returns, and sometimes with a vengeance. These kind of quick-fix fads also often deprive the body of a nutritional balance. Stick to a program that helps you to look *and* feel good. Look at the "Healthy Living" chapter for our guidelines.

THE MAKEOVERS

Sisters come in all shapes and sizes, and the most important thing is for us to feel comfortable with our own bodies. It's great to flaunt the curves of a full figure, but what do we do when there's just a little too much of us to love? Lisa, Joyce, Carol, and Natalie were four sisters in search of healthier diets, better fitness, and looking to lose a few pounds along the way. Carol and Natalie worked out with Sharone Huey, a professional trainer at the New York Sports Training Institute, and met with nutritionist Constance Brown-Riggs, who designed personalized weight-loss plans for their multifaceted makeovers.

Carol

Carol is like a lot of sisters in that she found it challenging to eat well and exercise while at the same time balancing a career as an accountant and raising her six-year-old son. With 183 pounds on her petite five-foot-two frame, Carol was motivated to get that weight off—and keep it off.

Sticking with a 1,500-calorie meal plan wasn't difficult for Carol, but cutting out the starches for a 1,200-calorie plan was a little tricky. She traditionally fried a lot of foods, and she never really worried about taking sec-

ond helpings at meals before. Now she moved to eating baked, broiled, and boiled meats instead of deep-fried delights. The new plan also meant smaller portions and smarter choices, like toast and a soft-boiled egg for breakfast instead of her usual pancakes and fried eggs.

When Carol first met with Sharone, her trainer, she described her goals as a flatter stomach, more muscle tone in her arms, and to lose a dress size. Because Carol was new to working out, Sharone decided to take things slowly, having her start with moderately paced walks and later incorporating light jogs and light weight training in the gym three days a

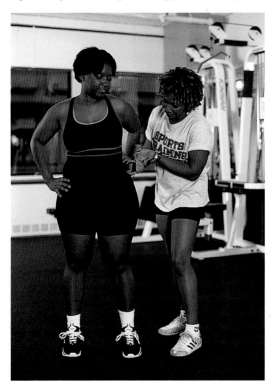

Left: Before. *Opposite:* With help from trainer Sharone Huey, Carol shed sixteen pounds and feels better than ever.

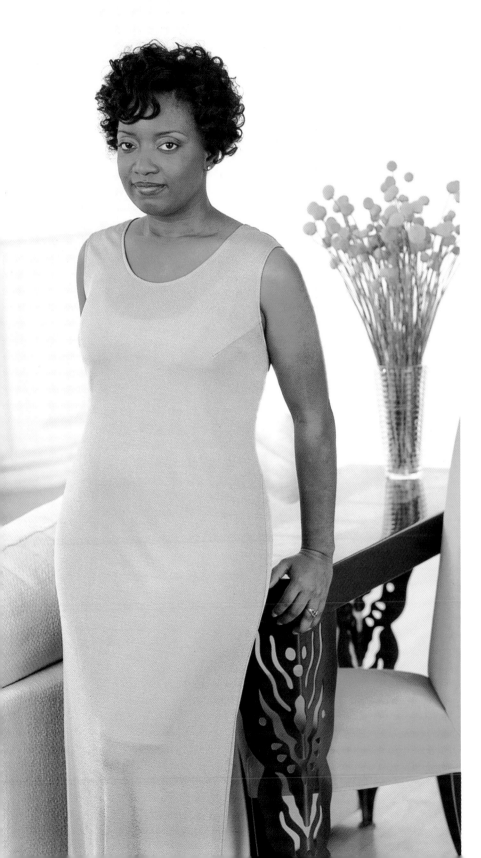

week. After she had a base of fitness from which to work, Carol began with ten minutes of cardiovascular work on the treadmill or bike before moving to forty-five minutes of weight training. This was followed by another hour of aerobics exercise, like walking, jogging, or stationary biking. Sharone also helped Carol start some abdominal work, like crunches. Carol worked out on her own during two more days in the week, walking about three miles around a track in her neighborhood.

After three months, the change was visible. Carol lost 16 pounds, ending up at 167. She went from a size 18 to a size 14, from a body fat percentage of 37 to 33, and lost 2 inches from her waist and hips. She felt so good about feeling good that she plans to continue to eat well and exercise at home with aerobics and hand weights, eventually heading to 155 pounds and a size 12. Most important, Carol understood the changes in her life as permanent and positive shifts in her health and fitness awareness, and finding a program she could stick with made all the hard work and sacrifice worthwhile.

Natalie

Natalie was a physical fitness buff in college, where she filled her weeks with four-mile runs, jumping rope, and sessions with a boxing trainer. After graduation, however, she moved to New York City and found herself spending late nights with friends in restaurants, laughing over french fries, macaroni and cheese, and other rich, overprocessed foods. A self-described "junk-food junkie," Natalie quickly put extra pounds on her five-foot-six frame—much of it on her hips.

Like Carol, Natalie found Constance's 1,500-calorie day a positive challenge to be met. It was difficult to cut out the fried food and the sweet treats, but Natalie had the hardest time letting go of her favorite food: bread. To spread her starch intake over the course of the day, she began with toast for breakfast in place of her usual bagel, and kept to eating serving-size portions of rice or a baked potato for the rest of the day. She also began planning her meals at home, where she could measure portions accurately and control the content of her meals to include ground turkey, chicken, tuna, steamed vegetables, and sweet potatoes cooked without salt or butter. Even on the rare occasion when she gave in to a sweet tooth craving, she limited herself to a small-size low-calorie candy bar.

At her first workout with Sharone, Natalie

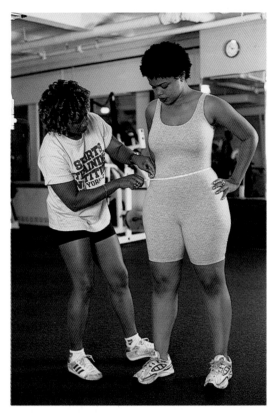

said she wanted to lose about twenty-five pounds and firm up her hips and buttocks. Because of the health risks associated with rapid weight loss and Natalie's personal history of losing weight slowly, Sharone cautioned her to expect to lose a more realistic ten pounds before starting her off on a program of three weekly workout sessions at the gym and two at home.

At the gym, Natalie spent forty-five minutes working with both free weights and weight machines, followed by an hour of cardiovascular work—aerobics, treadmill work, or riding the exercise bike. On her two workout days away from the gym, Natalie stayed active with aerobic exercise like running in the park near her home.

To shed even more pounds, Natalie dropped her daily caloric intake to only 1,000 halfway through the program. While this plan worked in the short run, without enough carbohydrates Natalie struggled in her workouts and suffered from a lack of energy for the rest of the day. After seeing a few extra inches disappear, Natalie was satisfied and knew that her future daily calories would have to total at least 1,200.

In three months, Natalie lost twelve pounds and her dress size went from a sixteen to a twelve. Her body fat percentage dropped as well, but the biggest change was in the way Natalie felt. With two inches gone from her chest and waist and several more lost in her hips, she was aware of having a slimmer face and feeling lighter. Another sign of her hard work and determination was evident in her arms and shoulders, as her entire upper body had become more defined from the light repetitions in her weight-training program. With those extra pounds gone and her interest in exercise rekindled, Natalie's plans to keep the weight off were destined to be a knockout success.

For Lisa and Joyce's health and fitness makeovers and training programs, see chapter 4.

Opposite: Before. *Right:* Natalie went from size sixteen to twelve and lost twelve pounds.

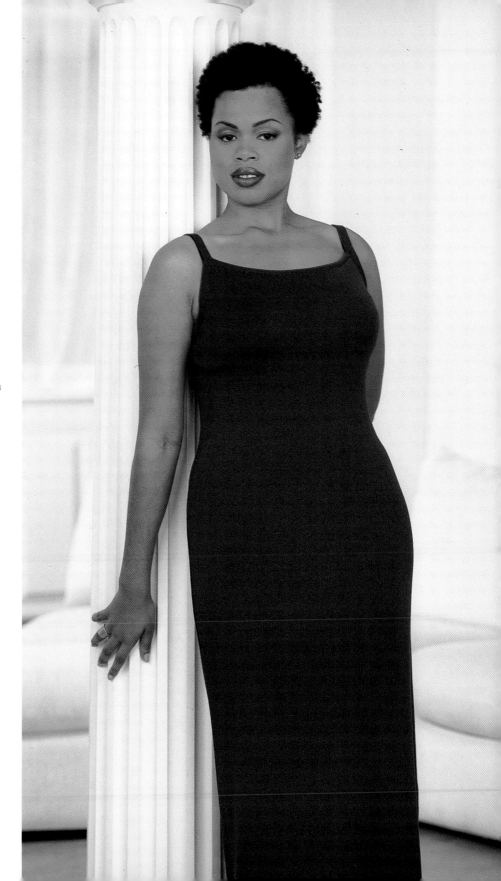

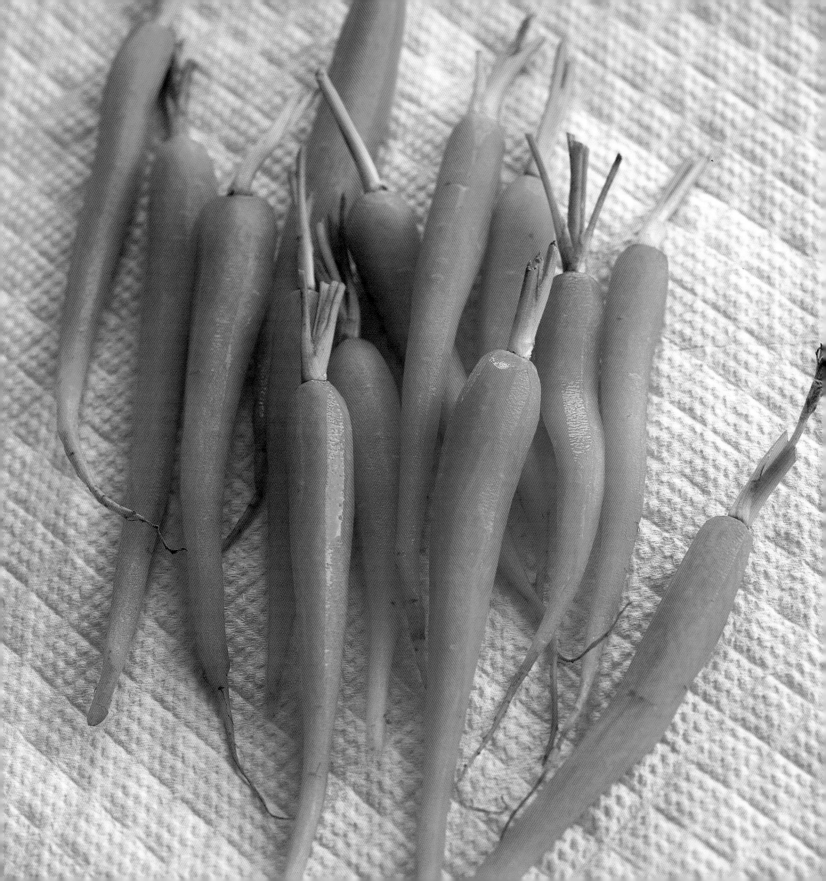

4 HEALTHY LIVING

MOST OF US KNOW GOOD HEALTH WHEN WE SEE IT. Whether it's a professional athlete, a complete vegetarian, or the elderly couple you see speedwalking each morning, images of healthy lifestyles are not uncommon. Yet many of us wonder how some healthy habits can fit into our lives. What's the big secret to good health?

There is no secret. Simply put, good health is a state of positive well-being. We actively stay well by taking good care of our bodies, living healthy lives, and committing to greater health awareness. With motivation and the right know-how, this awareness—and the feel-good fitness that comes with it—is available to each and every one of us.

In the same way that we approach our goals of emotional healing, spiritual strength, and outward beauty, we can pay attention to physical well-being. We can begin by praising ourselves for the kindness we've shown our bodies over the years, and understanding and forgiving ourselves for our past unhealthful practices. Now we're ready to go to the next level and live in the here and now!

If you're ready to make time in your life to get healthier, you are already on your way to enhancing—and extending—your life. And with support and your good example, the lives of those you love will benefit as well.

Below: Fresh fruit is delicious and nutritious. *Opposite:* Luscious strawberries are a rich source of vitamin C.

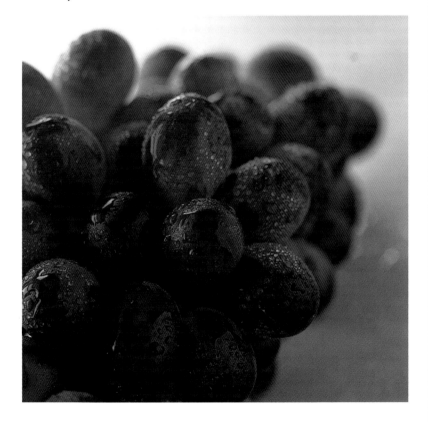

SELF-ASSESSMENT

How healthy are you?

- Do you feel good, physically and emotionally, most of the time?
- Are you rested when you wake up in the morning?
- Is your diet nutritious, with plenty of fruits and vegetables?
- Do you drink eight glasses of water a day?
- Do you exercise for at least twenty minutes, three times a week?
- Are you maintaining the proper weight for your build?
- Do you get regular medical checkups, even when you're feeling fine?
- If you have any medical conditions, are you sure you understand them and are clear about how to take care of yourself? Do you follow the advice of your health-care practitioners?
- If you take medication, do you take it as your health-care practitioner has prescribed, even after you feel better?
- Do you perform monthly breast self-examinations?
- Do you practice safe sex?
- Do you avoid smoking and illegal drugs?
- If you drink alcohol, do you drink in moderation?
- Are you able to relieve stress in constructive ways? Do you know about meditation, yoga, and exercise?

If you answered "yes" to most of these questions, you've got a good sense of the direction to move in for a healthier lifestyle.

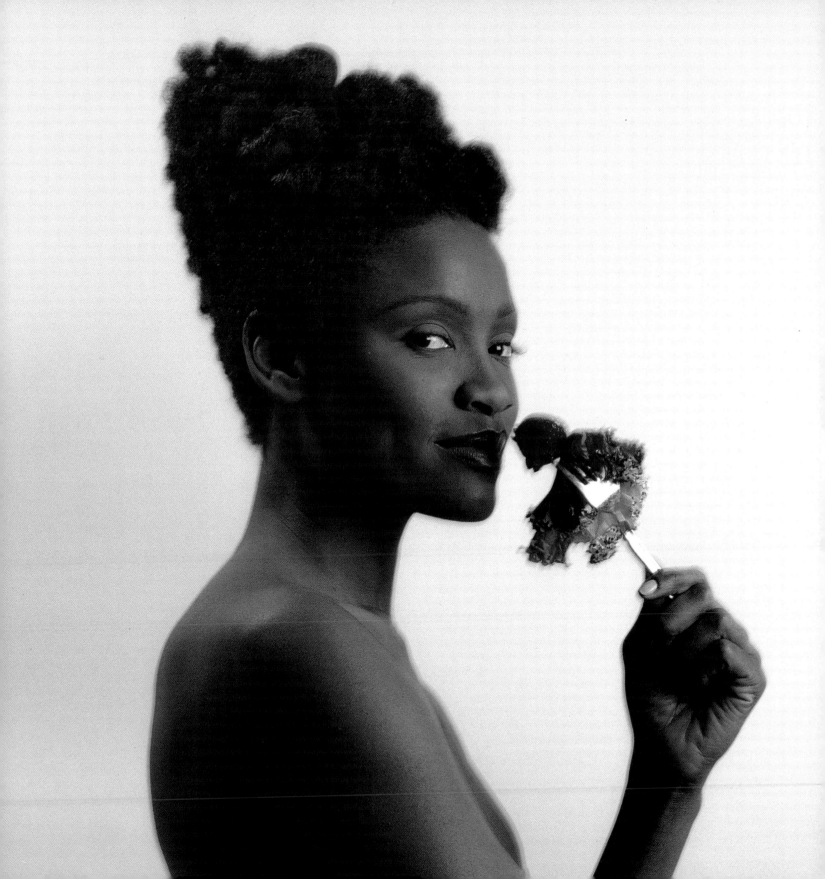

AN OUNCE OF PREVENTION

We can begin moving toward a healthier lifestyle by setting realistic goals. If you're one of those fortunate sisters who has already taken charge of her health, keep doing what you're doing! On the other hand, if you're like most of us, you know you need to make a change or two but just can't seem to find the time or energy to get started on that road to great health.

You need to pace yourself. You may be tempted to take a solemn vow to start exercising for an hour a day, cut out all the alcohol, and become a strict vegetarian—first thing Monday morning! Does this sound familiar? If there's even a chance that you'll be saying the same thing next month or next year, try taking it a little slower. Make a commitment to take the stairs up a few flights instead of using the elevator. Limit yourself to a glass of wine a day. Steam some broccoli instead of frying that steak. Go for it today, not Monday morning!

Quite a few ailments that people discover in their mature years actually begin to develop decades earlier, yet studies from around the globe suggest that through proper diet and a healthy lifestyle we have the power to cut down illnesses like colds and the flu, and dramatically reduce the risk of life-threatening diseases such as cancer. That's why it's impor-

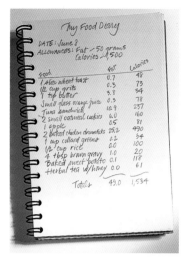

Above: It's a smart practice to keep track of your fat and calorie intake. *Opposite:* Nutritious foods supply vitamins and minerals.

tant to take proper care of yourself today. It's never too late to improve your health.

The prescription is more simple than you might think. Eat a nutritious, balanced diet, exercise regularly, drink eight glasses of water a day, limit or avoid alcohol, don't smoke, minimize stress, and get enough sleep.

For some folks, enough sleep means just six hours each night, while others require eight. Scrimping on slumber may appear to add precious hours to your busy day, but in the long run sleep deprivation can erode your concentration, weaken your memory, and make you more prone to anxiety, stress, accidents, and illness.

Get periodic medical checkups, even when you're feeling fine. A physician familiar with you and your medical history is well equipped to provide ongoing preventive care. Potential problems are often caught long before they become serious. Since many illnesses have few, if any, symptoms in the earliest stages, what you don't know *can* hurt you.

In between checkups pay attention to your body's signal that something might be amiss. Don't ignore a problem until it becomes impossible to ignore, as too many sisters and brothers do. Your grandmother was right: An ounce of prevention is definitely worth a pound of cure!

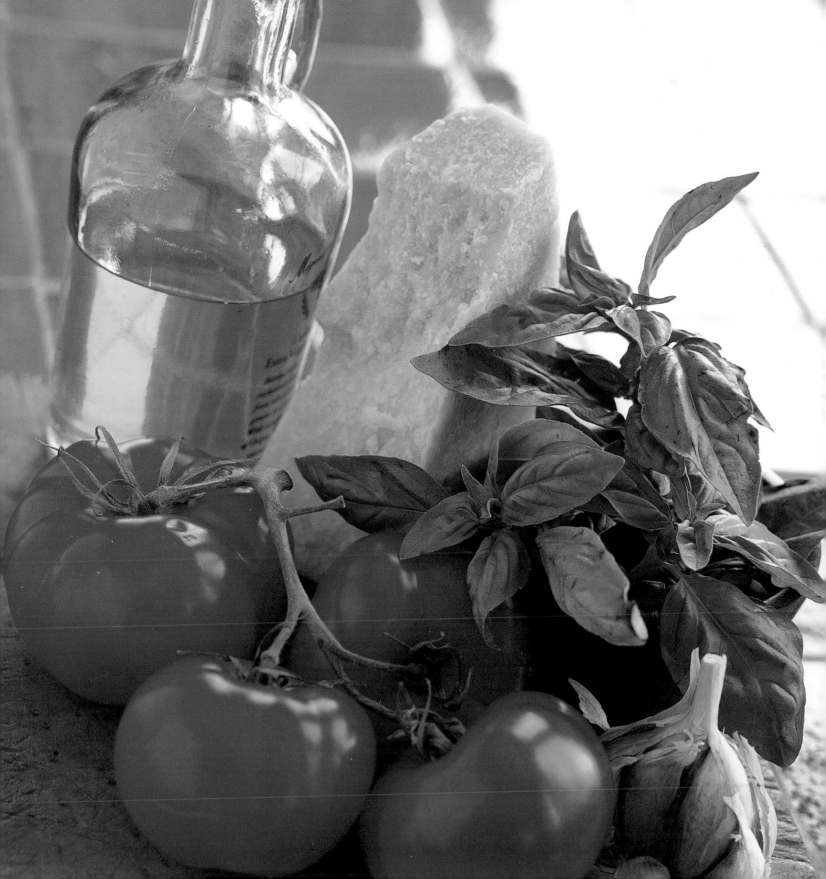

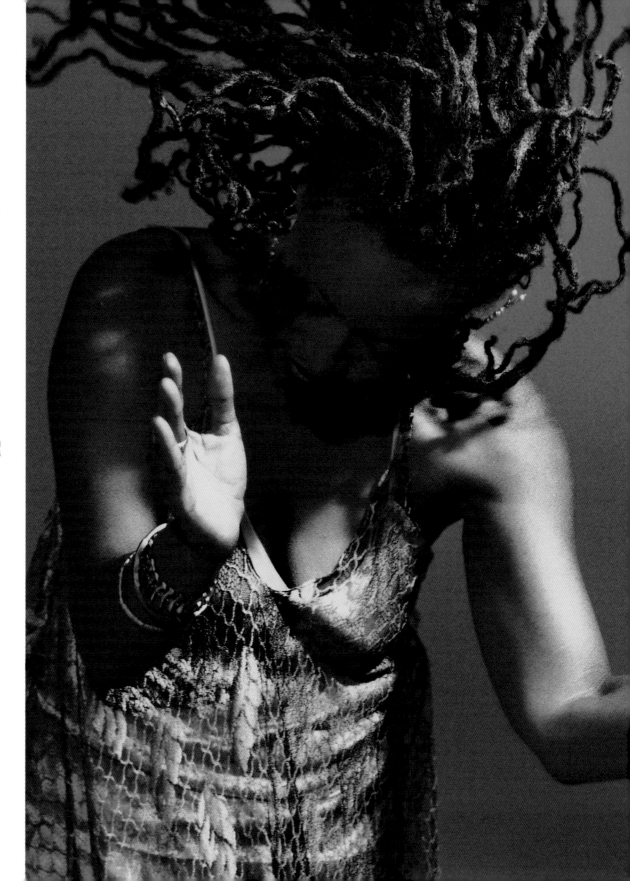

CASSANDRA WILSON

MY GRAND-
MOTHER WAS
ALWAYS OUT IN
THE WOODS
UNTIL SHE WAS
IN HER EIGHT-
IES. SHE WAS A
GARDENER
MOST OF HER
LIFE, BUT
SHE WOULD
SOJOURN
DAILY OUT IN
THE WOODS
WHERE SHE
WOULD GATHER
HERBS. SHE
UNDERSTOOD
HERBS.

EATING RIGHT

Most of us know plenty of sisters—and brothers—who can "burn" in the kitchen when it comes to cooking soul food. But as good as our traditional cooking tastes, it is rarely low in calories. Moreover, it is usually high in animal fat, salt, and sugar, which, when consumed in excess, can lead to health problems. The good news is that eating well doesn't have to mean depriving ourselves of tasty food. We don't have to give up all the foods we love. We simply need to learn how to prepare them in more healthful ways and satisfy ourselves with smaller portions. You might be surprised at how delicious food can be when cooked with your favorite herbs and spices instead of loads of salt and fat.

For optimum performance, your body needs certain nutrients that come from low-fat and low-cholesterol foods that are high in essential vitamins, minerals, and fiber. In other words, you can improve your present and future health by cutting down on or eliminating meat, butter and high-fat dairy products including cheese; limiting pastries, desserts, and sugar-sweetened drinks; and eating more whole grains, fruits, and vegetables.

Concentrate on unbleached and minimally processed foods—and the darker the better.

Below: Simply adding a salad at lunch can help you meet the daily goal of five servings of vegetables and fruits.
Opposite: Cassandra Wilson, jazz vocalist.

For instance, choose whole-grain bread and pasta, and brown rice instead of their whiter versions. Eat fresh or frozen fruits and vegetables instead of canned. Keep in mind that you destroy many nutrients in vegetables when you cook them until they're mushy, so try eating them raw or steam them so they keep their crunch. Fast foods (which tend to be high in salt, fat, and calories) and processed foods (such

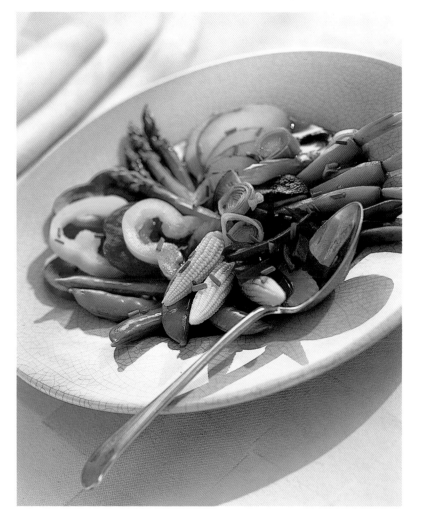

HEALTHY LIVING PLAN

Moderation is the key when it comes to healthy eating and dieting. For a daily intake of 1200 to 1500 calories, keep your meals within the following guidelines.

Food Group	Servings Per Day	Examples of One Serving
STARCH/BREAD	7	• 1 slice whole wheat bread • 3 ounces baked potato • ½ cup pasta • ⅓ cup rice
PROTEIN	5	• 1 ounce fish • 1 ounce lean beef • 1 egg • 1 tablespoon peanut butter • 3 ounces tofu or other soy product
VEGETABLES	4	• 1 cup raw vegetables • ½ cup cooked vegetables • 1 large tomato • ½ cup vegetable or tomato juice
FRUIT	4	• 1 medium fresh fruit • ¼ cup dried fruit • 15 grapes • ⅓ cup cranberry juice
DAIRY	2	• 1 cup milk • 8 ounces yogurt
FATS	3–4	• 1 teaspoon margarine, butter, cooking oil, or regular mayonnaise • 1 tablespoon regular salad dressing • 1 tablespoon nuts or seeds • 1 tablespoon cream cheese • 1 slice bacon
FREE FOODS	unlimited	• Vegetables (celery, cucumber, salad greens) • Condiments (mustard, hot sauce) • Seasonings (herbs, spices, soy sauce)

ONE DAY'S SAMPLE MENU

BREAKFAST

⅔ cup cranberry juice	2 fruit
8 ounces yogurt	1 dairy
½ cup oatmeal	1 starch

LUNCH

¼ cup tuna fish	1 protein
2 slices whole wheat bread	2 starch
1 teaspoon mayonnaise	1 fat
1 sliced tomato	1 vegetable
1 cup raw vegetables	1 vegetable
1 apple	1 fruit
12 ounces sparkling water	free

DINNER

4 ounces baked chicken	4 protein
3 ounces baked potato	1 starch
1 teaspoon butter	1 fat
½ cup steamed green beans	1 vegetable
mixed green salad	free
1 tablespoon salad dressing	1 fat
12 ounces sparkling water	free

SNACK

1 pear	1 fruit
3 cups plain popcorn	1 starch

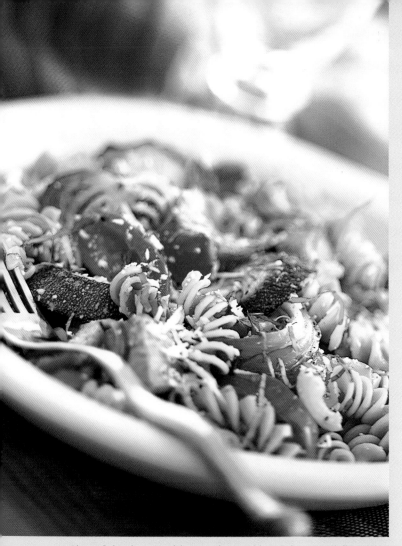

WHAT'S A SERVING?

Controlling your portions is essential to eating a nutritious diet and maintaining a healthy weight. As a general rule of thumb, one serving of food will fit into the palm of the average woman's hand. Note that a single piece of food is not necessarily a single portion. For instance, one fresh bagel can be five or six servings of your daily starch allowance, and one banana counts as two servings of fruit since it is high in carbohydrates.

Each of the following is an example of one serving:

1 medium fruit (such as an apple or orange the size of a softball)
$\frac{1}{2}$ cup of chopped fresh or cooked fruit
$\frac{3}{4}$ cup of 100 percent fruit juice
$\frac{1}{4}$ cup of dried fruit
1 cup of raw or $\frac{1}{2}$ cup of cooked vegetables
1 cup of raw leafy greens
$\frac{1}{3}$ cup of cooked beans (such as lentils, pinto, or kidney)
$\frac{1}{2}$ cup of cooked rice, pasta, or cereal
1 slice of bread
1 ounce of dry cereal
3 ounces of lean meat (about the size of a deck of cards)

CANCER-FIGHTING FOODS

New research has found that certain foods may contain cancer-blocking agents. Known as antioxidants, these naturally occurring chemical compounds protect the body's tissues from premature aging and degeneration. Vitamins C and E, beta-carotene, and selenium are the most potent. They are abundant in the following sources:

• the darkest green, yellow, and orange vegetables and fruits
• citrus fruit
• nuts and seeds
• seed oils

Remember, overcooking vegetables can diminish their cancer-fighting power.

Above: Spinach pasta with roasted vegetables. *Below:* A well-flavored, warm, and spicy chicken salad nourishes the soul, too.

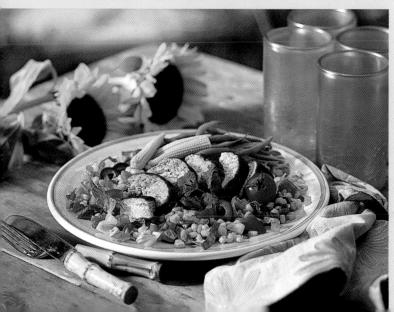

as frozen meals, lunchmeats, and packaged macaroni and cheese) should be kept to a minimum, if eaten at all.

An increasing number of sisters and brothers agree with some experts that the best road to health is through a vegetarian diet, one that excludes animal protein; yes, that means red meat, poultry, most seafood, and dairy foods. Vegetarian meals revolve around plenty of fresh fruits, vegetables, and whole grains. For the protein you would otherwise get from meat, you can load up on tofu or soy-based food, beans, peas, and sprouts. Nuts and seeds are also good protein sources, if kept to no more than two ounces. If you are not ready for a complete vegetarian diet, move to baked or broiled fish, which are better than red meat and poultry. Pork and shellfish should be avoided. Instead of cow's milk, cheese, ice cream, butter, and margarine, turn to the dairy-free and soybean-based versions of these foods. Soy products are highly nutritious and can mimic a variety of textures and flavors. Some nutritionists suggest that vegetarian diets should be supplemented with B-complex vitamins, especially B_{12} and brewer's yeast.

The U.S. Department of Agriculture (USDA) and the National Cancer Institute recommend that we eat at least five servings of fruits and vegetables each day. These plant foods are high in important nutrients such as vitamin C, beta-carotene, and folate and other

Above: Suzanne Douglas, actress.

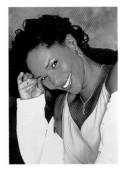

SUZANNE DOUGLAS AS BLACK WOMEN WE NEED TO MAKE A COMMITMENT TO TAKE CARE OF OURSELVES. YOUR HAIR AND SKIN ARE DIRECT REFLECTIONS OF WHAT YOU PUT INTO YOUR BODY.

B vitamins. The average American already gets about three daily servings, so simply adding a low-fat green salad to lunch and eating an apple as an afternoon or evening snack does the trick.

Your meals should include six to seven servings of minimally processed breads, cereals, rice, and pasta. The larger your frame and more physically active you are, the greater the number of servings you'll need. Consume two servings of dairy substitutes (or milk, cheese, or yogurt, if you want dairy) a day. If you're pregnant or between the ages of thirteen and twenty-five, you should have three servings. For protein, eat two or three daily servings of meat, beans, and nuts. Fat, oils, and sweets should be kept to a minimum.

Scientific evidence suggests that diet is the culprit in about one-third of the cancer deaths in the United States each year; obesity increases a person's risk of cancer, diabetes, heart attack, and other ailments. What you eat, and how much of it, really can make a difference.

THE LANGUAGE OF LABELS

Always read the "Nutrition Facts" label on the foods you buy. Notice the number of servings per package. Many foods seem low in calories until you realize that what looks like a single serving is described as two or one and a half

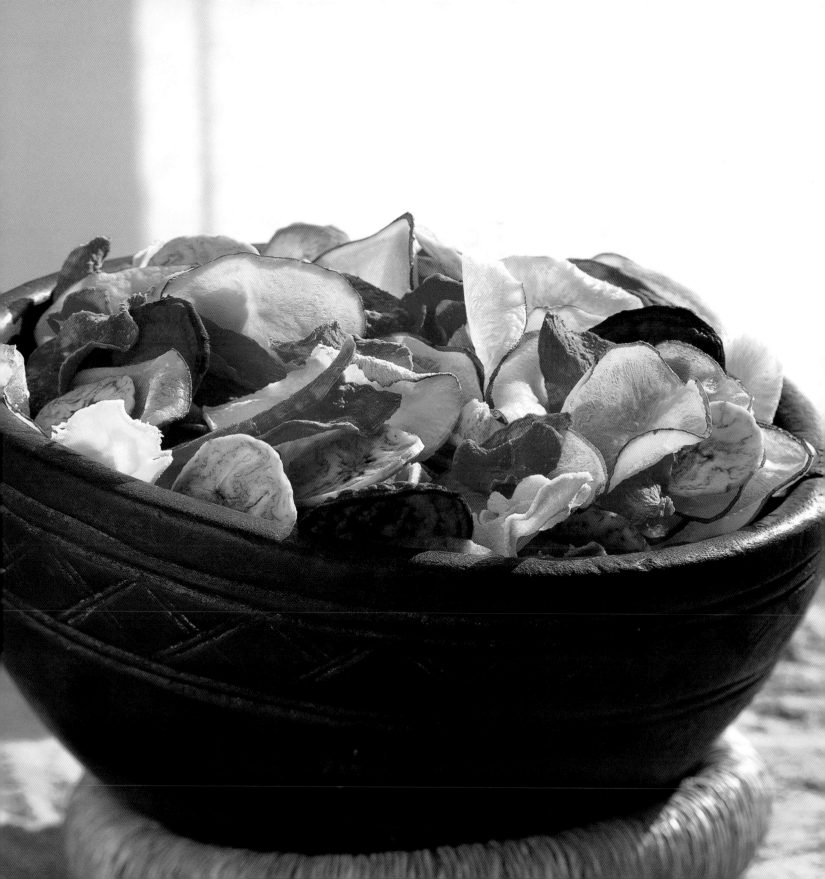

ESSENTIAL VITAMINS AND MINERALS

Vitamins (organic compounds) and minerals (inorganic) are crucial for maintaining normal growth and health.

Vitamin or Mineral	Benefits	Good Sources
VITAMIN A	Maintains health of skin, eyes, bones, teeth, and organs; important for new cell growth and fighting infection	Milk, eggs, liver; beta-carotene (in dark green and yellow-orange fruits and vegetables, such as spinach and carrots), which is converted to vitamin A in the body
B-COMPLEX VITAMINS (including folic acid)	Assists metabolism, helps prevent certain birth defects, helps to maintain the nervous and digestive systems	Brewer's yeast, meats, whole-grain cereals
VITAMIN C (ascorbic acid)	Creates and maintains connective tissue, fights bacterial infection, aids production of blood cells, antioxidant	Fresh fruits (especially citrus) and vegetables (especially green peppers and potatoes)
VITAMIN D	Aids the heart by absorbing calcium and phosphorus, promotes healthy teeth and bones	Eggs, fish, fish liver oil, and dairy products
VITAMIN E	An antioxidant that aids heart functions and vascular health, prolongs life of red blood cells	Most vegetable and seed oils, wheat germ, eggs, nuts, leafy vegetables, blackstrap molasses
VITAMIN K	Promotes coagulation of blood, promotes healthy functioning and longevity of the liver	Kelp, spinach, kale, egg yolk, fish liver oil, blackstrap molasses, yogurt
CALCIUM	Builds strong bones and teeth, calms nerves and aids insomnia, normalizes blood clotting, regulates muscular contraction, minimizes PMS symptoms	Milk products, green vegetables, whole grains, salmon, sardines, peanuts, soy products
IRON	Forms hemoglobin (red blood cell pigment that transports oxygen), increases resistance to stress and disease	Red meat, liver, fish, eggs, fruits, vegetables, breads, cereals, brewer's yeast
MAGNESIUM	Aids metabolism and functioning of nerves and muscles, antistress mineral	Nuts, whole-grain foods, dry beans, green vegetables, soy products
PHOSPHORUS	Promotes health of bones, teeth, cells, nerves, and kidneys	Meat, fish, poultry, eggs, whole grains, seeds, and nuts
POTASSIUM	Aids nerves, muscles, and heart function and blood's mineral balance, helps lower blood pressure	Vegetables (especially green leafy), oranges, whole grains, potatoes, bananas
SELENIUM	Along with vitamin E, it aids metabolism, body growth, and fertility	Bran, broccoli, onions, tomatoes, tuna, and wheat germ
ZINC	Aids digestion, metabolism, general growth, and functioning of reproductive organs and prostate gland, promotes development and healing of new cells	Brewer's yeast, beans, nuts, seeds, wheat germ, fish, and meat

servings on the label. Remember that "low fat" and "low calorie" are not the same thing. Low-fat cookies, for example, may be high in sugar—and calories—to compensate for the loss in flavor from the decrease in fat. Choose foods with the least amounts of saturated fats, sugar, and sodium.

VITAMINS AND MINERALS

Americans spend millions of dollars each year on vitamin supplements. Ideally, your nutrients should come from your diet, not a bottle of pills. Yet getting enough of the necessary vitamins and minerals consistently may be difficult, even with the healthiest eating habits. Taking multiple-vitamin supplements can be added insurance.

Certain vitamins may help guard against specific illnesses. Research has shown that foods rich in vitamin C (including citrus fruits, strawberries, tomatoes, broccoli, and both green and red peppers) promote healthy gums. Women whose diets are high in vitamins C and E, beta-carotene, and folate also seem to reduce the length and severity of their cold symptoms. If you come down with a cold, think as much about what you can take out of your diet as you do about what you put in; some studies have shown that even a tablespoon or two of sugar can significantly reduce the immune system's ability to fight off illness.

Be sure to consult your doctor or nutritionist before taking extra doses of individual vitamins. Megadoses of some supplements—for example, vitamin A—can have serious side effects.

DIETING

Forget those quick fixes—the powdered meal-replacement drinks, the miracle pills, the low-cal frozen dinners. Patience is the key. A healthy diet teaches you how to lead a healthy life—not just the constant calorie cutting and counting that leaves you feeling deprived. Slimming down gradually, developing healthier eating habits, and exercising regularly will not only ensure that you are losing fat instead of lean tissue, but it will also help you make a lasting lifestyle change.

DEALING WITH DOCTORS

Not all doctors are created equal, so it's important to find a good one with whom you feel comfortable, especially when it comes to choosing a primary care physician and a gynecologist. "Comfortable?" you may ask, "While you're naked in front of a virtual stranger who could tell you something you really don't want to hear?" Visiting a doctor can be unsettling, but there are things you can do to make the experience a positive one.

When you're looking for a physician, shop

around. You wouldn't buy the first car you check out or the first dress you take from the rack, so why feel compelled to stick with the first doctor you see if you weren't completely satisfied?

Studies have shown that many doctors give men and women different medical attention. Many times, women's health concerns are interpreted as mere hysterics or exaggerated complaints. During the examination, be sure to ask the physician to clarify anything you don't understand about any ailments, treatment options, and possible side effects of medication. Speak clearly and openly with your doctor. No matter how embarrassed you may be, it doesn't help you one bit to keep your "business" to yourself if talking about it could provide a clearer picture of your health.

Even after you find an excellent doctor with a wonderful bedside manner, it is normal to feel some degree of unease or to be overwhelmed by everything the physician has told you. Before each visit, prepare a list of questions to take along so you won't forget anything you want to ask. Take notes while the doctor is talking, or ask for a copy of the doctor's notes after the exam. Also, you have every right to have a copy of anything and everything in your medical file. If you ever switch doctors, don't be timid about asking that your records be sent to another physician.

Right: Dr. Deborah Simmons closely examines a patient's skin.

JADA PINKETT SMITH EATS CHICKEN AND FISH AS A SUBSTITUTE FOR RED MEAT TO BUILD PROTEIN.

LENA HORNE ATTRIBUTES HER GOOD HEALTH TO AVOIDING CAFFEINE AND NICOTINE.

JACKIE JOYNER-KERSEE DRINKS LOTS OF WATER EVERY DAY TO KEEP HER BODY HEALTHY AND FREE OF TOXINS.

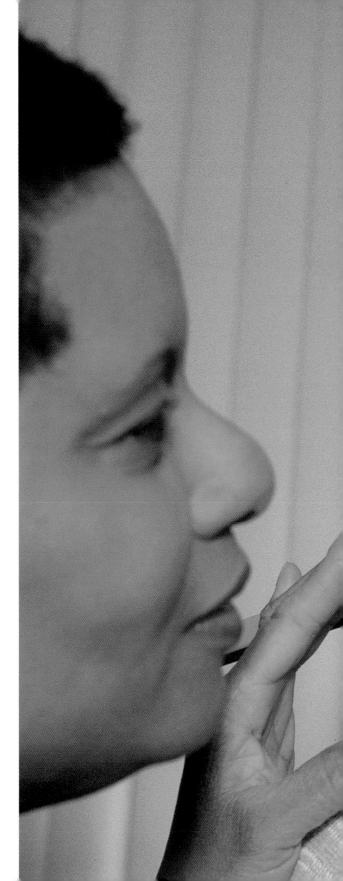

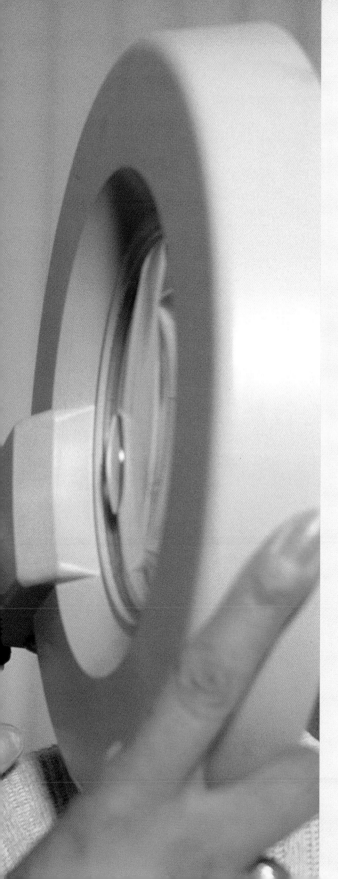

THE DOCTOR IS IN

Remember to schedule regular visits for preventive checkups. Most of us should see the following doctors.

PRIMARY CARE PHYSICIAN (family practitioner, internist, or general practitioner) *once a year.* During a routine physical, expect the doctor to check your height and weight, pulse, blood pressure, breathing, and your body temperature. The doctor will also examine your eyes, ears, nose, and throat, perform bloodwork, and discuss any immunization updates you should consider, such as vaccines against tetanus, hepatitis B, or influenza (the flu).

GYNECOLOGIST *once a year.* Gynecologists are female reproductive system specialists who may also serve as primary care physicians. Obstetrician/gynecologists (OB-GYNs) are trained to deliver babies as well. During a pelvic exam, this doctor looks for abnormal growths such as fibroids, cysts, malformed organs, and indications of infection. Regular visits will detect chlamydia and gonorrhea, two precursors to pelvic inflammatory disease (PID), which can cause severe pain and infertility. The gynecologist will also examine your breasts for potentially cancerous lumps. If you are not sure how to perform your monthly breast self-examinations correctly, ask her. Be prepared for a rectal exam, along with a Pap smear to check for infections and cancerous or precancerous cells that might indicate cervical cancer. If you are sexually active and do not use condoms 100 percent of the time, you should be checked for other sexually transmitted diseases (STDs). Survival improves with early diagnosis—and fortunately, more Black women are making the choice to take these simple precautions.

OPHTHALMOLOGIST OR OPTOMETRIST *every two years, or more often after age forty.* An ophthalmologist is a physician who diagnoses and treats eye disorders (including glaucoma and cataracts), measures vision, and prescribes corrective lenses. An optometrist, an OD (doctor of optometry), measures vision, prescribes glasses or contact lenses, and screens for eye disorders.

DENTIST *every six months.* Along with brushing at least twice a day (after breakfast and before bed) with a soft toothbrush and flossing at least once daily, periodic dental cleanings and checkups can prevent gum disease, an ailment more common among African-Americans than the rest of the population. At best, it can cause chronic bad breath and bleeding gums. At worst, it could cause your teeth to loosen and fall out. Every three to five years, you should have dental X-rays to detect any hidden damage to teeth or jawbones.

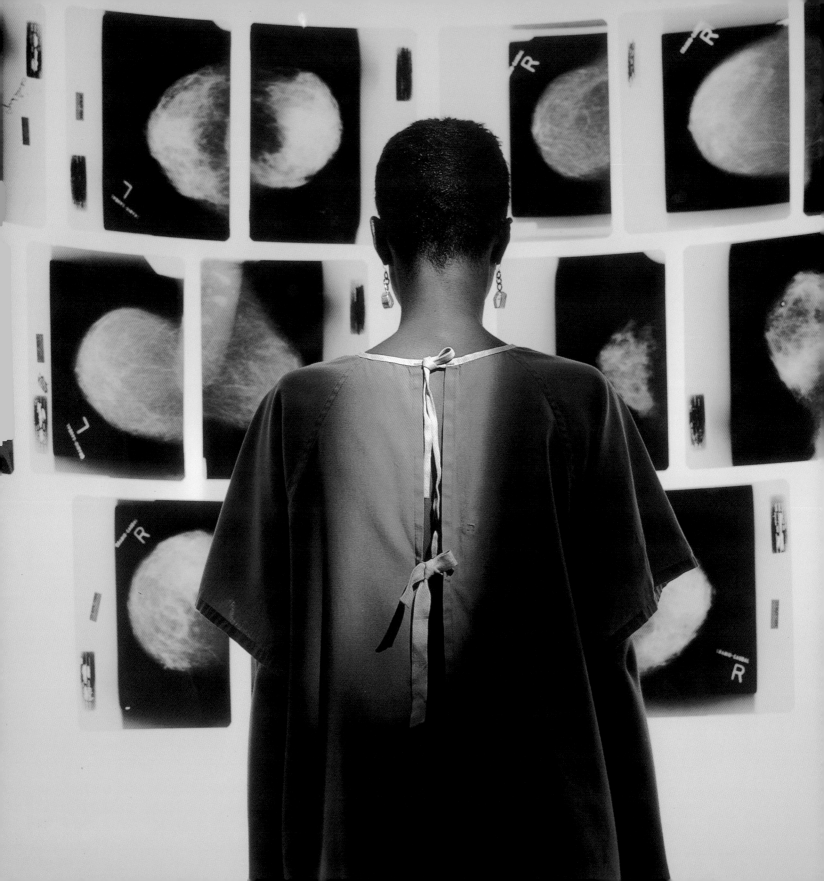

TEST TIME

When you go for your routine medical visit, you may undergo a variety of tests. Certain tests and some procedures will be completed while you are at the doctor's office, while the results of others may not be known for a week or so. Here are the most common medical tests:

Test	To Detect	When
MAMMOGRAM	Breast cancer	A baseline mammogram between ages 35 and 40. Every one or two years from age 40 to 50, and annually after that. Women with family histories of breast cancer should have the earliest and most frequent mammograms.
PAP SMEAR	Cervical cancer and infections such as herpes, vaginal warts, yeast, and other sexually transmitted diseases (STDs)	Yearly, or every two years for all women aged 18 and older and for younger women as soon as they become sexually active
CHLAMYDIA SCREENING	Chlamydia, an STD that can cause pelvic inflammatory disease (PID) and infertility but often has no symptoms until the advanced stages	Periodically for sexually active women
SCREENING FOR OTHER SEXUALLY TRANSMITTED DISEASES	STDs including syphilis, gonorrhea, HIV/AIDS	If you have symptoms or are at risk
BLOOD CHEMISTRY PROFILES	Anemia, leukemia, high cholesterol, diabetes, hypertension, liver and kidney diseases, thyroid problems, and other disorders, HIV/AIDS	Annually or as per doctor's recommendation
BLOOD SUGAR LEVELS	Diabetes	Routine throughout life, especially during pregnancy
URINALYSIS	Diabetes, bladder or kidney infections	Annually
GLAUCOMA TEST	Elevated eye pressure	Annually after age 40
CHEST X-RAY	Pulmonary diseases, heart disease	Baseline, then according to physician's directions
TB SKIN TEST	Tuberculosis	Annually
SIGMOIDOSCOPY OR COLONOSCOPY	Colon and rectal cancer	Initial test between ages 50 and 55, then every three to five years. Earlier if you have colon or rectal problems or a family history of colorectal cancer.

ALTERNATIVE HEALING

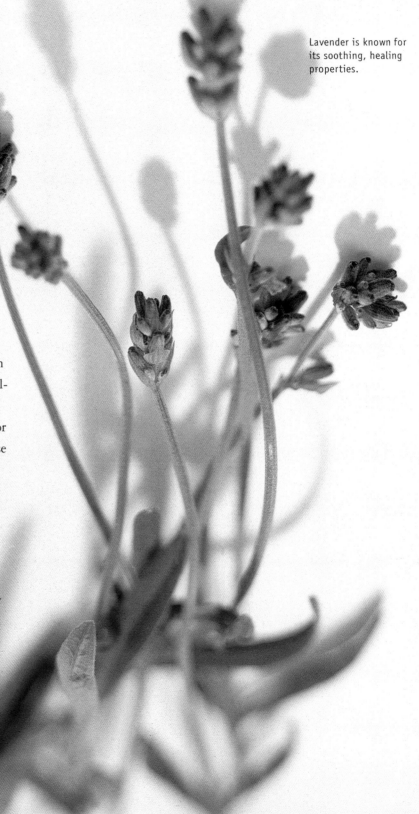

Lavender is known for its soothing, healing properties.

The line between mainstream and alternative healing is becoming less defined. In 1993, the health insurance industry began subsidizing the costs for successful treatment of heart disease that involves dietary changes, meditation, visualization, and exercise.

Today, more African-American women are moving beyond conventional Western medicine in search of greater health and healing. In increasing numbers, we are seeking out herbalists, chiropractors, acupuncturists, massage therapists, and other practitioners of natural or holistic medicine. Sometimes we do so because we feel that traditional health care has failed us. Other times, we simply want to broaden our options for treatment.

Because herbs, the predecessors of modern medicine, can have powerful (though sometimes slow-acting) effects, you should seek expert advice before taking any. Be extra careful to consult with a physician or licensed herbalist if you are pregnant or nursing.

COMMON HEALING HERBS

Herb	Use	Form
ALOE VERA	Laxative; soothes burns and ulcers	1/4 cup liquid gel, morning and evenings, or capsules for internal use; leaf pulp for external use
BLACK COHOSH	Treats symptoms of PMS and menopause	Tincture or 1/2 cup loose tea steeped in hot water and strained
CHAMOMILE	Settles gastrointestinal upsets; relieves menstrual cramps; a natural sedative	1 cup tea, 2 to 3 times daily
CRANBERRY	Helps prevent urinary infection	2 to 3 cups unsweetened juice, on 1 or 2 capsules or tablets daily of standardized extract
ECHINACEA	Stimulates immune system; helps fight cold and flus	Tea, tablets, capsules, or 2 or 3 drops tincture from leaf or root, 3 to 4 times daily
FEVERFEW	Eases migraines, chronic headaches, anti-inflammatory	2 capsules or powder, or 1 to 2 drops tincture
GARLIC	Lowers cholesterol and triglyceride levels; antibacterial, antiviral, and antifungal	2 to 3 cloves, capsule, or tablet daily
GINGER	Relieves morning sickness and stomachaches; relieves cramps	Ground ginger, shaved fresh ginger, powder, beverages, decoction, or tincture
GINKGO BILOBA	An antioxidant; increases blood circulation and oxygenation; improves memory	Tablets, capsules, extract, tincture, or loose tea
GINSENG	Increases stamina	Tea, tablets, or tincture
GOLDENSEAL	Antiseptic; used with echinacea to fight colds and the flu, anti-inflammatory	Capsules, tea, or tincture
LAVENDER	Relieves nausea, calms	Tea or tincture
LICORICE	Soothes ulcers, relieves stomach upset, anti-inflammatory	Tea or standardized extract
RED RASPBERRY	Helps treat canker sores, cramps, spasms, hot flashes; strengthens the uterus	Tea

HEALTH 911
SPECIAL CONCERNS

Allergies

When the body mistakenly produces antibodies to "protect" itself from normally harmless substances, allergies result. Do you find yourself sneezing, wheezing, and dabbing your runny nose and itchy, teary eyes when pollen is in full force or when animals or dust mites are around? These symptoms suggest that you have allergies. Whether you have seasonal hay fever or year-round allergies, you may not have to depend on fatigue-inducing antihistamines for relief.

In addition to changing your immediate environment, try boosting your immune system by eating lots of fruits and vegetables, drinking plenty of water, exercising regularly, getting enough rest, and reducing stress. To supplement traditional medical therapies, some people have relieved allergies by taking extra vitamin C each day. Consider consulting a homeopath who, after a detailed review of your symptoms, will choose a specific homeopathic remedy to get your sneezes under control.

Asthma

Affecting almost ten million Americans, asthma is an inflammatory disease of the lungs that affects a disproportionate number of African-Americans. In fact, we're three times as likely to die from the disease than whites.

Although the exact cause of the disease is unknown, it can be triggered by air pollution, cigarette smoke, dust, mold, animal hair, pollen, stress, exercise, dairy products, and even cockroaches. Characterized by fits of wheezing, coughing, shortness of breath, and tightness in the chest, asthma attacks can usually be kept at bay with proper medication and preventive efforts.

Lupus

Almost twice as common among Black women as it is among white women, systemic lupus erythematosus—lupus—is a chronic disease that causes the immune system to attack the body's tissues instead of protecting them from disease. The cause of lupus remains unknown, but doctors think it is linked to genetics and other factors such as infections, antibiotics, ultraviolet light, and extreme stress. Because lupus affects people in different ways and in different parts of the body, it's extremely difficult to diagnose. Nevertheless, there are warning signs and symptoms such as swollen joints, persistent fatigue, chronic fever, unusual hair loss, skin rashes, hypersensitivity to the sun, and nausea or other stomach discomfort. A cure for lupus has yet to be discovered, but early detection, medication, and attentive care can keep the symptoms manageable.

GYNECOLOGICAL CONDITIONS

Pregnancy, fibroids, premenstrual syndrome, and menopause are frequent topics of discussion among Black women, as they well should be. When we have quality medical information and act on what we've learned, we bring ourselves closer to the positive state of well-being we are aiming for.

Fibroids

At least 50 percent of African-American women of childbearing age have fibroids, though many don't know it. These noncancerous uterine tumors, also known as myomas, are about two to three times more common among Black women than white women. Heredity, a high-fat diet, and being overweight all seem to increase the risk.

Fibroids never cause problems for some women; after menopause, they usually shrink and sometimes disappear. For others, symptoms such as heavy menstrual bleeding, painful intercourse, frequent urination, or infertility require medical attention.

Fibroids can often be managed through drugs or noninvasive means. Some sisters have found that these growths shrink and symptoms disappear as a result of acupuncture, taking herbs, following a vegetarian diet, and/or adopting relaxation techniques to reduce stress.

Hysterectomies are often performed to solve the problem, but many doctors say that removal of the uterus is rarely necessary. During a myomectomy, the fibroid is surgically removed, leaving the uterus intact. However, fibroids sometimes return. If your doctor suggests a surgical procedure, get a second opinion; surgery of any kind should be a last resort.

Premenstrual Syndrome (PMS)

You've got a killer headache and cramps. Your face is breaking out, you're bloated, and you're moody. Welcome to premenstrual syndrome—PMS. Yes, girl, it's those two weeks before your period is due, but there may be hope for you after all.

Recent research has found that calcium can greatly relieve the symptoms of PMS. Use soy products, eat lots of leafy greens, or ask your health-care practitioner about taking calcium supplements. Ginger also may reduce cramps, as will cutting down on salt, eliminating caffeine, and eating low-fat foods. Vitamin B_6 supplements taken for three days before PMS symptoms start has also been suggested, but do this only under expert supervision since megadoses of B_6 can be harmful.

Consuming five or six small meals a day instead of three large ones might be effective as well, particularly in smoothing out mood swings. Eat a good balance of complex carbohydrates and moderate amounts of protein. Finally, reducing your stress through exercise, meditation, and relaxation can help as well.

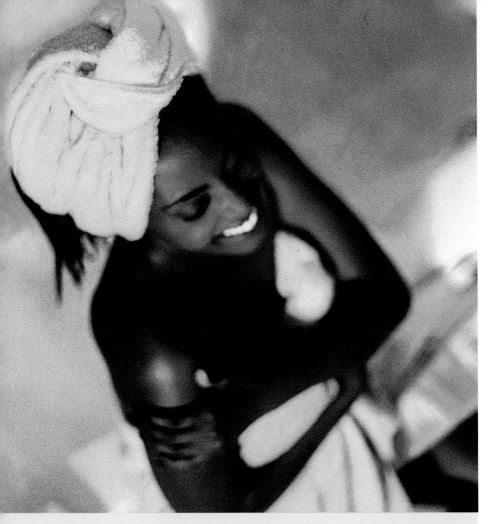

THAT-TIME-OF-THE-MONTH BATH

Whether your premenstrual symptoms are severe or mild, this one can help get you through "the visit." Some people swear it eases the cramps, mood swings, headaches, cravings, and bloating that often come with menstrual periods. Use these essential oils in your bath.

5 drops lavender
2 drops geranium
2 drops grapefruit
1 drop clary sage
2 tablespoons canola, olive, or almond oil

Mix the oils and stir them into a warm bath. Soak and relax. Use in the days leading up to your cycle for best results, and remember you will get through this monthly period, like all others.

Pregnancy

Planning for a healthy pregnancy is important for sisters. Studies show that pregnancies of Black women are at greater risk for adverse outcomes. Whether with birth defects like fetal alcohol syndrome (FAS), low-birth-weight babies, or infant mortality, Black people are regrettably overrepresented.

Start taking care of your body several months before you plan to get pregnant. If you drink excessively, smoke, or use illegal drugs, get help to quit. If you are overweight, start dropping pounds. Improve your diet. Gaining too much weight during pregnancy could cause you to develop dangerous complications such as gestational diabetes, toxemia, or high blood pressure. Sign up for a prenatal exercise, aerobics, or childbirth class.

Begin prenatal care as early as possible, and be sure to keep all appointments with your doctor. Ask her about prescription drugs that could cause birth defects. Get a physical to make sure your body's in good shape. Ask your obstetrician's advice about prenatal vitamins, especially folic acid prior to conception as a means of lowering the risk of serious birth defects. Read baby books. The more you know, the more at ease you'll feel during the pregnancy.

Menopause

Menopause is the beginning of a new and exciting, free phase of your life. You'll no longer

MENOPAUSE: SYMPTOMS AND TREATMENTS

Symptom / Condition	Alternative Remedies	Possible Side Effects	Conventional Treatments	Possible Side Effects
HOT FLASHES, NIGHT SWEATS	No caffeine or alcohol		Estrogen (HRT)	Breast pain, headache, risk of breast and uterine cancer, gallbladder disease
	High soy diet	Allergic reaction		
	Vitamin E	Toxic at high levels	Estrogen and progestin (HRT)	Risk of breast cancer, gallbladder disease, weight gain, menstrual bleeding
	Herbs:			
	black cohosh	Nausea		
	dong quai	Sun sensitivity		
	licorice	High blood pressure		
	Natural progesterone cream (from wild yam)	Abrupt stop causes menstrual bleeding		
VAGINAL DRYNESS	Lubricants, sex		HRT	See above
	Vaginal cream (from wild yam)	Unknown	Vaginal estrogen cream	
FORGETFULNESS	Reading, mental exercises		HRT	See above
	Herbs:			
	ginseng	High blood pressure, nervousness, bleeding		
	gingko biloba	Headaches		
LOW SEX DRIVE	Exercise, stress reduction		Estrogen with testerone (HRT)	Acne, weight gain, liver disease
	Herbs:			
	damiana	Blocks iron absorption		
	saw palmetto			
MOOD SWINGS, ANXIETY	Exercise, meditation		Antidepressants	Addiction
	Herbs:		Therapy	
	St. John's wort	Sun sensitivity		
	motherwort	Menstrual bleeding		

have to worry about birth control. You'll never have to buy yourself another box of tampons. And best of all, you're wiser than ever.

Once your periods have stopped for a year, it's a pretty safe bet that you have reached menopause. This usually happens around age fifty. Some women ease into menopause with little difficulty. Others experience a host of symptoms, including hot flashes, vaginal dryness, interrupted sleep, fatigue, confusion, moodiness, and dry hair, skin, and nails. You can alleviate some symptoms of menopause by following a well-balanced diet that is rich in calcium (and soy foods such as tofu), avoiding alcohol, exercising regularly, and reducing stress.

Some women may be candidates for hormone replacement therapy (HRT). The hormone estrogen can alleviate many symptoms of menopause, as well as head off osteoporosis, cardiovascular disease, and memory loss. However, due to the increased risk of uterine cancer associated with taking estrogen alone, it is often prescribed in conjunction with progesterone. Taken together these hormones can aid the transition to mature womanhood. Ask your doctor what she thinks, as these therapies have side effects and are not recommended for women with a family history of breast cancer, blood clots, unexplained bleeding, or fibrocystic breasts. A combination of traditional and alternative treatments might work best for you.

OUR MOST COMMON LIFE-THREATENING ILLNESSES

Whether the reasons are hereditary, environmental, or behavioral, some medical conditions disproportionately affect our community. Of these, the leading causes of death among African-American women are heart disease, hypertension, and strokes; cancer of the breast, lung, or colorectal region; HIV/AIDS; and diabetic complications.

Heart Disease

There is a misperception that women do not suffer from heart attacks as much as men do; this is largely because their symptoms are misdiagnosed and many women wait longer before seeking medical attention during cardiac arrest. Make sure your doctor keeps an eye on the health of your heart, especially if you are postmenopausal. Among Black women, the rate of death from heart disease—cardiovascular disease—was a whopping 69 percent higher than among white women, although the rate has been steadily declining over the past decade.

Arteriosclerosis (hardening of the arteries) and high cholesterol are among the most dangerous of the conditions leading to heart disease. About one out of every four African-Americans suffers from hypertension, and we develop high blood pressure earlier in life. Moreover, we often have high cholesterol levels and are believed to smoke more than other women.

More than 50 percent of African-American women are overweight. High-salt, high-fat diets contribute to our higher rates of hypertension, which is a major cause of strokes (blockage of the blood vessels that supply oxygen to the brain), kidney failure, and heart failure.

Strokes

Strokes, or cerebrovascular accidents (CVAs), hit 500,000 Americans a year, leaving nearly a third of that number dead and the remaining often seriously impaired. The majority of strokes are triggered by blood clots blocking the oxygen supply to the brain, while others are caused by high blood pressure destroying small blood vessels, leaving them to bleed into the brain.

The risk of strokes increases with high blood pressure, high stress levels, smoking, and excessive alcohol consumption. Medical conditions such as sickle cell disease, lupus, diabetes, as well as aging are also known to put you in the danger zone for strokes.

Play it safe and take care of yourself. Keep your weight and diet under control, lower your stress level, meditate, and stay in close contact with your doctor.

Cancer

Breast cancer is second only to *lung cancer* as a leading cause of death of women in this coun-

try. Every year, 180,000 women are diagnosed with breast cancer, and about 46,000 die from it. Overall, Black women have a lower survival rate, 65 percent after five years, compared with 79 percent among white women. However, under age forty-five, we have a higher survival rate. Now, more Black women are having breast examinations and mammograms, and giving up cigarettes, but breast and lung cancers are still among the leading causes of the illnesses and deaths of our sisters. *Cervical cancer* is about three times more common in Black women in comparison with white, but can be detected by regular Pap smear tests and cured if caught early. *Colorectal cancer* (cancer of the large intestine) is the third leading cause of cancer deaths in women, and the survival rate among Black women has been lower than that of white women for nearly twenty-five years. Early detection would certainly increase our chances of survival.

HIV and AIDS

HIV (human immunodeficiency virus) is the virus that triggers AIDS (acquired immunodeficiency syndrome), the leading killer of Black women and men between the ages of twenty-five and forty-four. HIV is most frequently transmitted through unprotected sex and IV drug needle sharing with an already infected person, and a cure for AIDS has yet to be found. Treatment and prevention programs

COMMON LIFE-THREATENING ILLNESSES

Disease/Condition	Risk Factors	Warning Signs and Symptoms
HIV/AIDS	Multiple sex partners, intercourse with a bisexual man, unprotected vaginal or anal intercourse, history of sexually transmitted disease, IV drug use, blood transfusions between 1977 and 1985	Swollen lymph glands, fatigue, chills, fever, night sweats, chronic diarrhea, yeast infections, and sudden weight loss
CANCER	Positive family history, cigarette smoking, excessive alcohol consumption, high-fat diet, use of oral contraceptives, overexposure to the sun	Unusual lumps, moles, or "pimples"; pain; unexplained fatigue; sudden weight loss; swollen glands; blood in urine, stools, or phlegm
DIABETES	Positive family history, obesity, unhealthy diet, excessive alcohol consumption, lack of physical activity, delivering newborn babies over nine pounds	Slow-healing cuts, bladder or yeast infections, frequent urination, excessive thirst, unexplained weight loss, constant hunger with little weight gain, advanced symptoms include blurred vision, unexplained drowsiness, and numbness or tingling in hands and feet
HEART DISEASE	Positive family history, high cholesterol, high blood pressure, high-fat diet, cigarette/tobacco smoking, physical inactivity, stress, obesity, excessive alcohol consumption, excessive red meat consumption	Pain, tightness, or a burning sensation in the chest, especially on the left side; sudden neck, jaw, or arm pain, especially on the left side; heart palpitations; sudden sweating or nausea; shortness of breath; swelling of the legs; fatigue
STROKES	High blood pressure, smoking, birth control pills, atherosclerosis	Body numbness; headache on one side of the head; difficulty speaking, seeing, walking, or swallowing; dizziness
HYPERTENSION (HIGH BLOOD PRESSURE)	Obesity, stress, high-fat and –salt diet, excessive alcohol consumption	Usually no symptoms initially, but headaches, changes in mental activity, and blurred vision may follow later

Opposite: A healthy lifestyle today can mean peace of mind later in life.

are rapidly improving, but infection rates in our community have skyrocketed.

Diabetes

The number of Black people with diabetes has tripled since the 1960s, making it the fourth leading cause of death (by disease) in our communities. Among Black women, this condition has reached what the American Diabetes Association has called epidemic proportions. One out of every four Black women over age fifty-five has diabetes. More than half of us who have it don't even know it because the symptoms appear gradually and can be mistaken for ordinary signs of aging.

Diabetes is not only dangerous in and of

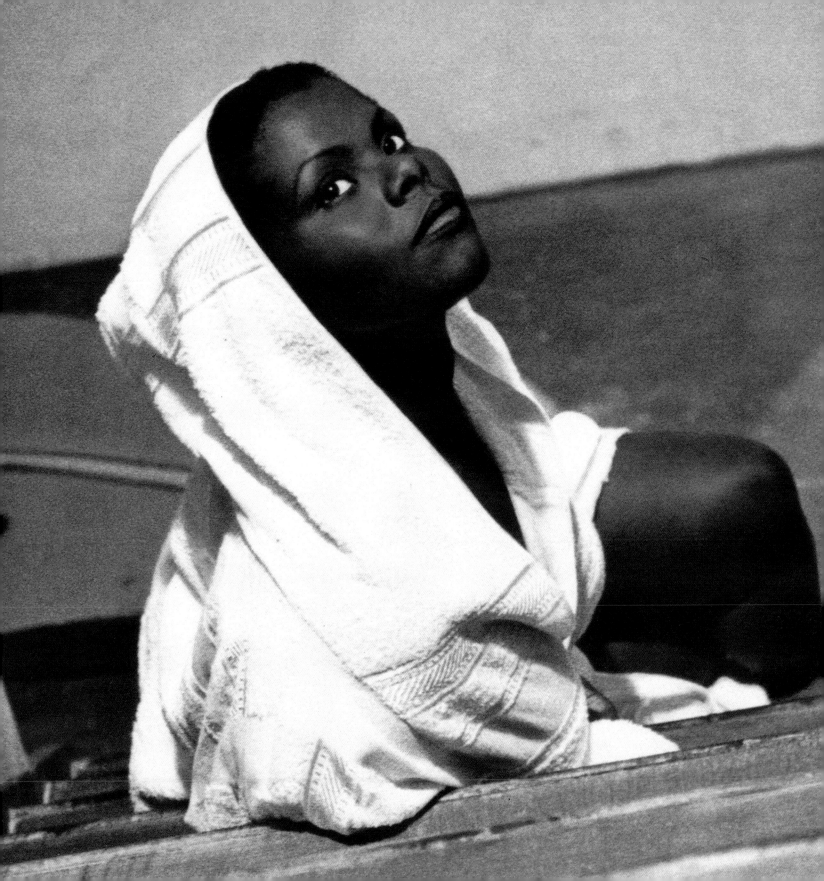

EXPERT ADVICE

"You can learn how to incorporate the foods you love into your meal planning in a healthy way. See what you currently eat and how you can work that into healthier eating habits." —Constance Brown-Riggs, nutritionist, New York

"When taking charge of your health, ask yourself, 'If I have a medical problem, do I understand it and am I following the prescribed regimen? Am I informed? Have I drawn from both traditional medicine and holistic methods to heal myself?'" —Dr. Opella Finley Oliver, family practitioner, Detroit

"Don't abuse your mind or body with drugs, alcohol, or unhealthy sex. Try to eliminate the negatives from your life. A negative attitude will do you more harm than a bucket of chitlins." —Dr. Andi Coleman, obstetrician/gynecologist, Detroit

"Women are still not aware of how barrier methods—condoms and diaphragms—help prevent sexually transmitted diseases." —Dr. Lewanzer Lassiter, obstetrician/gynecologist, Chicago

"Eat green, drink green (vegetable juices daily), and meditate on green grass. Beets, kale, broccoli, spinach all boost your immunity. Turnips are good for calming nerves, as well as strengthening joints, bones, and teeth. Put at least 50 percent live (raw or lightly steamed) foods in your system. You'll have more energy." —Queen Afua, holistic practitioner, Brooklyn, New York

"A consistent regimen of exercise may be more important than any medication you may take." —Dr. Carlyle H. Miller, internist/gastroenterologist, New York

"When beginning a fitness program, don't be discouraged if you don't see results immediately. Be persistent." —Ryan Gentles, personal trainer, Zion Physical Fitness, Brooklyn, New York

itself, but its complications can also lead to blindness, kidney failure, and neurological problems. Complications of diabetes, as well as gestational diabetes in pregnancy, are more dangerous for Black women than for others. We are 80 percent more likely than white women to develop diabetes during pregnancy, and our overall maternal mortality rate is much higher—fives times that of white women.

Luckily, diabetes can be helped by taking insulin, aerobic exercise, and eating a healthy diet to maintain blood sugar levels. Your doctor can give you a special diabetes testing kit to use at home, as well as advise you on how and when to test your blood sugar.

THE MAKEOVERS

Many women want to eat healthfully and slim down at the same time, but with all the crash diets out there, we need a little direction to get started. *Essence* enlisted a nutritionist and two personal trainers to help Lisa, Joyce, Carol, and Natalie fight the battle of the bulge.

For this phase of the health and fitness makeover, Joyce, Lisa, Carol and Natalie met with Constance Brown-Riggs, a Long Island, New York–based dietitian. At their first meeting, Constance guided the women through a nutrition questionnaire exploring their eating patterns and attitudes about food. She also asked them to provide sample food diaries so she would be better able to assess their eating habits.

Constance shared her ideas about understanding healthy eating as a positive lifestyle change, and she carefully explained that she didn't consider her meal plans "diets," which so many of us have tried with little lasting success. She said that one important step is taking the "I can't's—I can't eat this food, I can't eat that food"—out of conventional weight-loss attitudes. Instead, Constance asked, What can you do? What foods can you eat? What changes can you make in your diet?

Constance designed meal plans for the four women based on a daily total caloric intake, which was their goal weight multiplied by ten. For Lisa, Carol, and Natalie this meant 1,500 calories a day, while Joyce aimed for 1,200 calories a day. Constance told them to expect a gradual drop of one to two pounds a week. Halfway through the program, the women tried for 1,000–1,200 calories a day to increase their short-term weight loss. The main figure Constance used to determine how much weight each woman lost was their body mass index (BMI).

For each day, Constance's plan broke down to seven servings of starch, five of protein, four of fruit and vegetables, four of fat, and two of dairy. This food could be spread out over up to six medium-size meals, a tactic Constance said deals with hunger and maintains a high metabolism better than eating one or two big meals during the day.

Although it sounds easy on paper, the biggest challenge for Joyce, Lisa, Carol, and Natalie came when Constance told them a big-serving secret: weight loss is all about portion. A serving size of rice is not a cup-size mound, but rather $\frac{1}{3}$ cup, which fits easily in the palm of the hand. The sisters were also shocked to learn that a serving size of meat should be no bigger than a deck of playing cards, and that one bagel could take up almost all of a day's allotment of starch! By keeping food diaries, Joyce, Lisa, Carol, and Natalie were better able to track the foods they were eating—and stay more aware of their eating habits, too.

For the other half of their weight-loss program, the four women consulted personal trainers. Joyce and Lisa met with personal trainer Ryan Gentles from Zion Physical Fitness in Brooklyn. Ryan discussed gym workouts and gave advice on at-home exercise. He designed low-impact cardiovascular routines including treadmills, exercise bikes, free weights and weight machines, aerobics, and walking and jogging.

The weight-loss program was more than a walk in the park, but after three months Joyce, Lisa, Carol, and Natalie had shed some unwanted pounds and were enjoying the benefits of being more fit and firmer.

Lisa

Many sisters experiencing weight gain during pregnancy are often unable to get rid of the extra pounds after the delivery. Lisa was a proud new mother, but between her love of cakes and other baked goods and her hearty appetite for soul foods like barbecue chicken, she knew her body was in need of a tune-up.

Because Lisa was breastfeeding, Constance was sure to keep Lisa's meal plan at 1,500 calories a day so that the weight-loss program wouldn't interfere with her breast milk production. Yet even with that health concern in mind, Lisa was able to make the kind of changes in her diet that translated to better eating habits and safe, gradual weight loss. A breakfast of tea and toast replaced a ham-and-fried-egg sandwich, and salads began to make frequent appearances at lunchtime. Instead of meals of greasy, overprocessed takeout food, Lisa prepared dinners of fish or baked chicken with rice and vegetables.

Like the other sisters in the weight-loss program, however, the biggest adjustment for Lisa was getting used to eating smaller portions. With extra support from her husband, who was also looking to slim down, she still prepared many of the same dishes as she had before, except that now she had leftovers after the meal. Together, Lisa and her husband discovered that they didn't have to overeat to be satisfied.

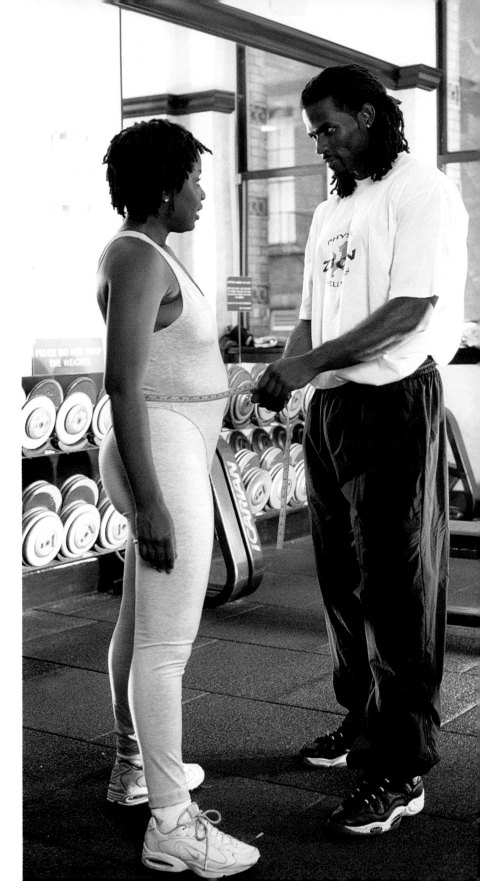

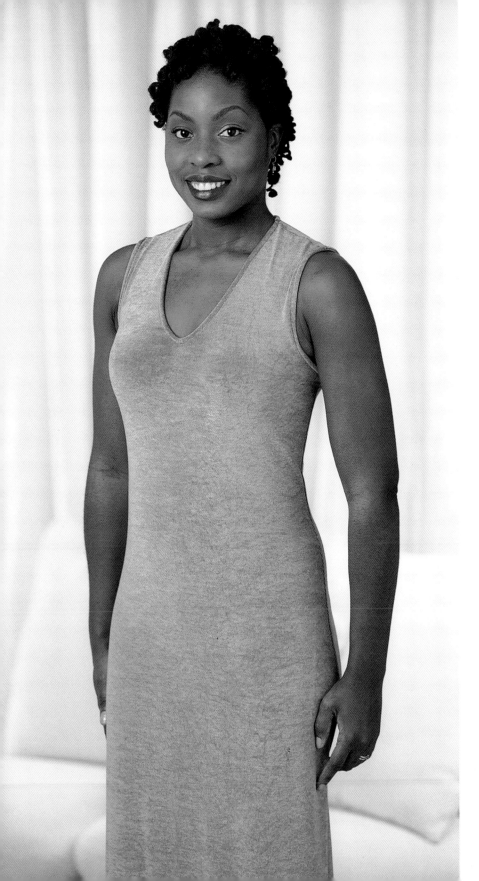

When Lisa met with Ryan Gentles of Brooklyn-based Zion Physical Fitness, she told him her goal was to lose ten to fifteen pounds, as well as to firm up her stomach and buttocks, which had rounded out of shape during pregnancy. Ryan designed a schedule in which Lisa worked out in the gym three days a week, starting with a warm-up and followed by a forty-five-minute cardiovascular workout on the treadmill, exercise bike, or with calisthenics. Ryan rotated these exercises to give variety in the workout, and added a weight routine at the end to tone and strengthen her body. To finish the session, Lisa pushed through a set of two hundred crunches! On each of her two training days outside of the gym she took thirty-minute jogs and did a hundred crunches.

With the demands of her job and a new baby, Lisa had a hard time keeping up with both Ryan's workouts and Constance's meal plans. Still, after three months, Lisa was thrilled with her results. She had dropped ten pounds from her five-foot-three frame and had gone from a size ten to a size six. Most important, her BMI came down from a 25.7 to a healthy 23.9. While she was unsure if she'd be able to maintain such a rigorous training program in the immediate future, she was confident that she would continue her healthy new diet and stick to her new rule: no seconds!

Opposite: Before. *Left:* Lisa is a slimmer, healthier new mom after following trainer Ryan Gentles's workout plan.

Joyce

Joyce grew up always being able to eat as she pleased, but as she moved into middle age, she found herself gaining weight and losing energy. With her blood pressure going up, her doctor told her she had to begin to lose some of her newly acquired pounds. Since she was between jobs, she had plenty of time on her hands—and no excuse not to get fit.

Constance started Joyce off on a meal plan of 1,200 calories a day. Because she was anemic, Joyce improvised a little—adding a little extra protein in her diet while cutting back on her daily allotment of starches and sugars. Before working with Constance, Joyce said she would eat three starches in a meal without even thinking about it, especially since she loved fried chicken, potato salad, and macaroni and cheese so much! Yet after she started the weight-loss program, she focused on eating fish and ground turkey, fruit, and salads with fat-free dressing. She also began to shy away from red meat and started cooking with lighter products and much less fat. Another healthy habit Joyce picked up was drinking lots of water, which helps weight loss by filling you up and clearing out your body's systems. Joyce started each day with a glass or two in the morning, kept a tall glass near her in the afternoon, and guzzled another two before bed.

At the gym, Joyce told Ryan that she

Right: Before. *Opposite:* Healthy eating habits and moderate exercise helped Joyce lose fifteen pounds.

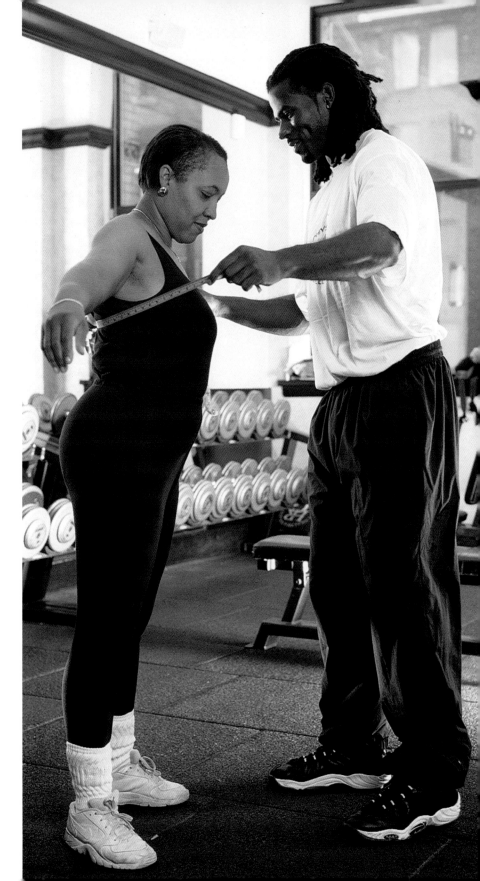

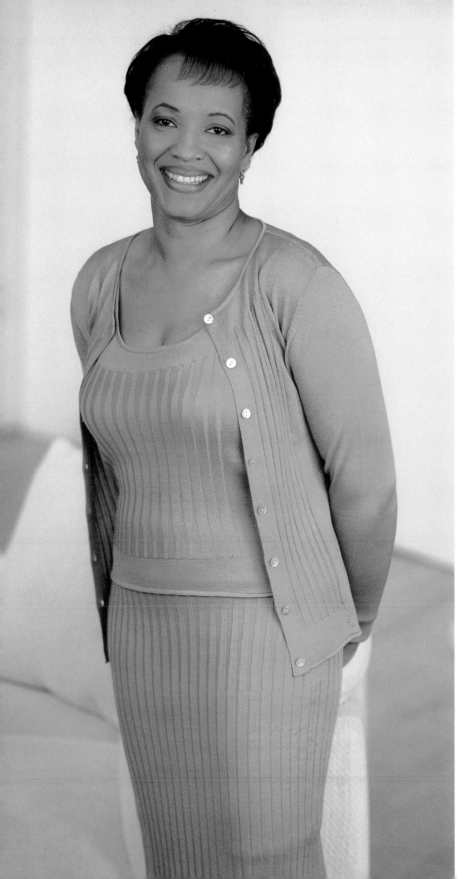

wanted to use working out to accent her eating plans and maintain a healthy body. Because she was new to working out, they began slowly, with Ryan stressing the importance of warming up before moving her on to a half hour of light weights, followed by forty-five minutes of cardiovascular work such as a quick-paced walk on the treadmill. Joyce finished each session with a set of crunches. On her own twice a week, Joyce spent up to an hour taking walks and doing sets of crunches.

Joyce's motivation and gung-ho attitude paid off. She shed away fifteen pounds and her BMI went from 28 to a healthy 25. After she found herself slipping into sizes six and eight when she used to squeeze into tens and twelves, Joyce was almost afraid she'd need to buy a new wardrobe! Yet the biggest change for her came in the form of a positive new attitude—she knew the new Joyce was here to stay.

See Carol and Natalie's health and fitness makeovers and training programs in chapter 3.

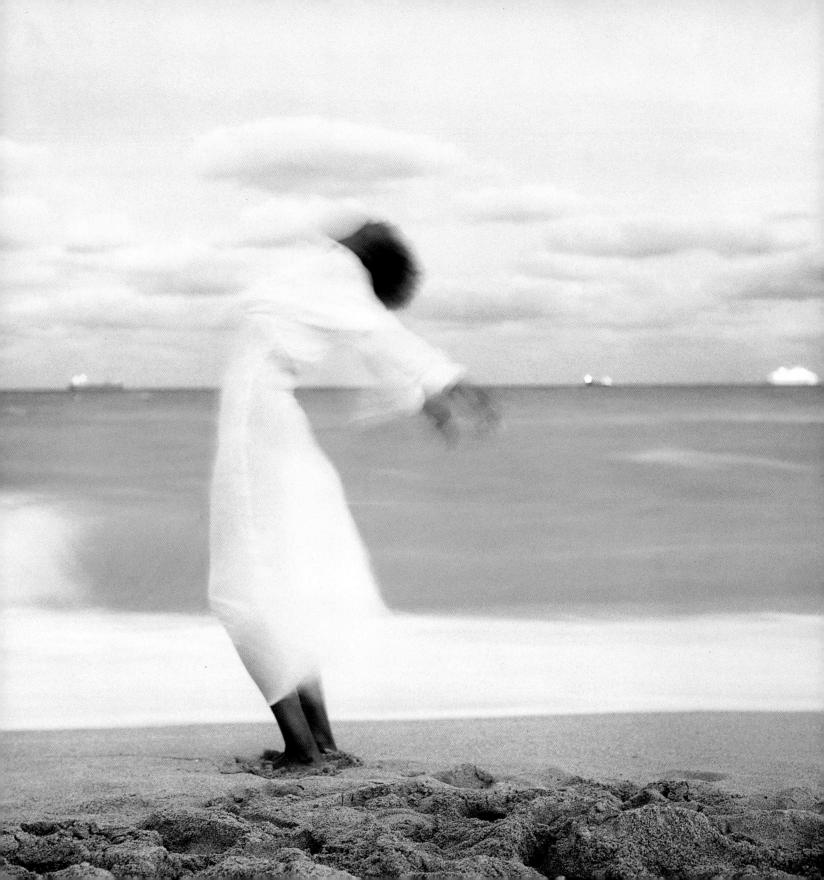

5 MENTAL WELLNESS

LAUGHTER IS AN AMAZING GIFT AND AN ENDURING TREASURE. We use it to celebrate our success, communicate our joy, and even to get us through times of misfortune. Our laughter lets everyone around us—including ourselves—know that everything is A-O.K., or soon will be.

There are other ways of expressing a peaceful state of mind. Whether with quiet time spent alone with a good book, or at a sleepover party with a few sisterfriends, we know that whatever we do to preserve our mental wellness—that peace—is just as important as taking care of our body and soul. Mental wellness is about living with a general sense of well-being. You're at peace with yourself and know that you are a worthy human being, deserving of love. You have positive relationships with others, and you know how to give and receive love. Your life is in balance. When you encounter difficulties, you allow yourself to experience the full range of normal emotions. You have the ability to see yourself through the hard times, and give yourself the freedom to enjoy the good times. You trust yourself and are confident that you will do your best in any situation. You always have. You know when to ask for help, and when it's best to go it alone.

Getting our lives in balance may take some doing, but we're worth it. And in taking this journey, we are bound to bump into some pain along the way. But let's not be discouraged or run from it. Pain is a signal that something in your life isn't working. Deal with it head on. Start by taking stock and sifting through your life to see what is working and what isn't. Bear in mind that this isn't about judgment—there isn't a soul out there whose life couldn't use a little fine-tuning, no matter how well things seem to be going. Begin taking inventory of your mental wellness with this self-assessment.

SELF-ASSESSMENT THE SIX MOST COMMON CHALLENGES TO MENTAL WELLNESS

DEPRESSION
- Have you lost interest in many things that were important to you?
- Do you often feel anxious or irritable?
- Do you often feel sad?
- Have you been questioning your self-worth or had lingering feelings of guilt?
- Have you noticed changes in your appetite, sleep patterns, or ability to concentrate?

COPING WITH LOSS
- Are you recovering from the loss of a loved one?
- Does this feeling of loss dominate your thoughts?
- Do feelings of regret and/or abandonment sometimes overwhelm you?

RELATIONSHIPS
- Do you solely depend on your personal relationships for your own happiness?
- Do you see an unhealthy pattern with the partners and relationships you choose?
- Are you or have you been in an emotionally or physically abusive relationship?

ADDICTIONS
- Do you crave cigarettes, caffeine, illegal drugs, or sex?
- Do you drink too much? Have you suffered a "blackout?"
- Do you gamble excessively?

EATING DISORDERS
- Do you go on food binges?
- Do you eat, or stop eating, when you're upset?
- Do you starve yourself, even make yourself vomit or take laxatives, to try to control your weight?

MONEY
- Would you have a hard time coming up with a figure for your total monthly bills?
- Do you spend next month's paycheck before you get paid or depend on your credit cards for most purchases?
- Do you frequently borrow money to make ends meet?

If you answered "yes" to one or more questions in any category, we know you will find comfort and solutions in this chapter that will help you to restore peace and balance to your life.

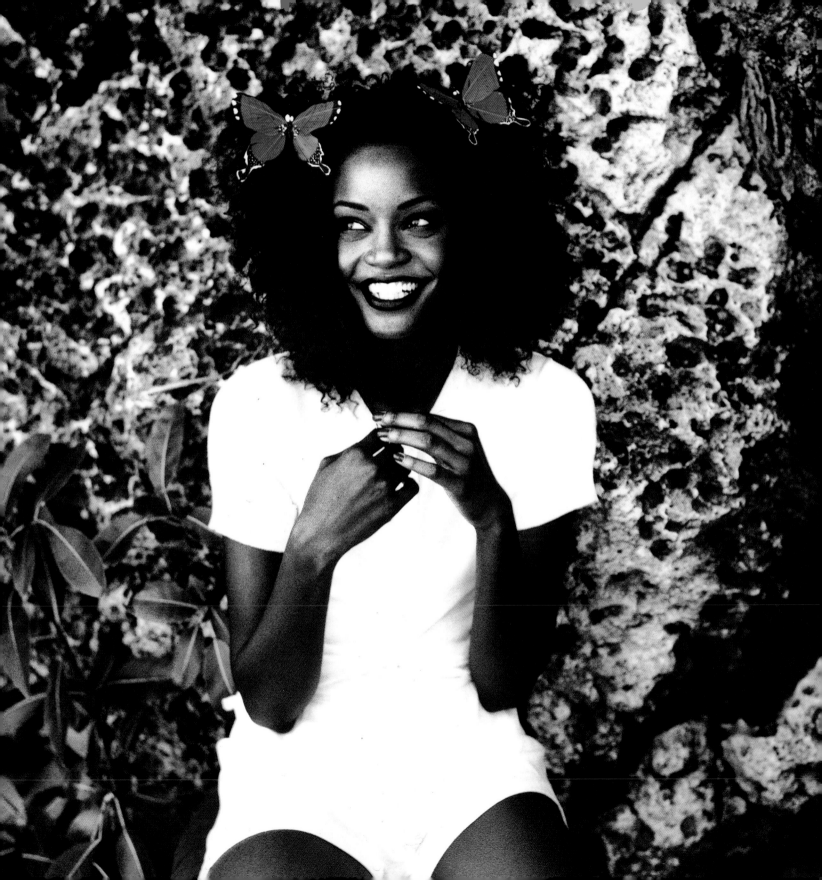

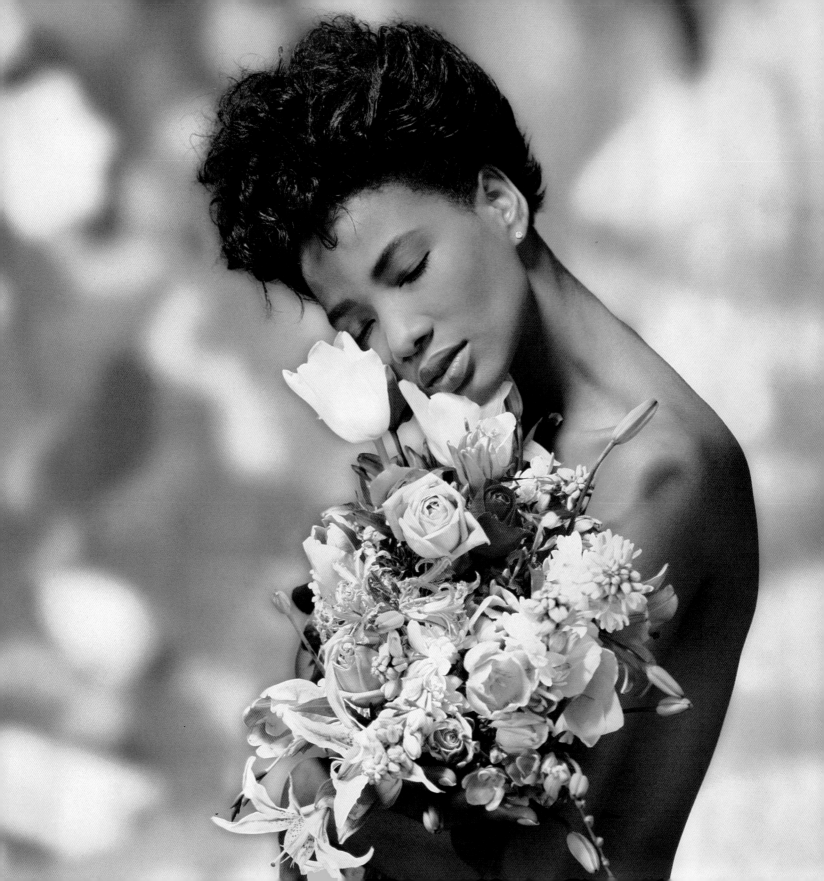

THE BLUES: HOW TO COMBAT DEPRESSION

MOODINESS

You're having one of those days when nothing seems to go right. You burst into tears in the ladies' room. You're wondering, What's wrong with me?

Everyone has moods. There are things that will upset you, and there will be times when you'll feel down in the dumps. But moods, by definition, are transient.

Some moods may be biological in origin. The changes in hormonal levels that cause premenstrual syndrome (PMS), for example, can make you feel as though you've temporarily lost your mind. The good news is that PMS is predictable. If you track your cycle by keeping a record in your calendar, you can predict when you'll be most vulnerable to sudden attacks of moodiness and can do something about it. Rest, exercise, and pampering yourself go a long way toward easing your crankiness during this time.

Depression, on the other hand, can range from mild to severe. While severe or recurrent depression may require professional interven-

Opposite: Embrace the beautiful things in life.

tion, mild depression and bad moods can be worked out on your own. There's a lot that you can do to improve your mood.

• REMIND YOURSELF THAT "THE BLUES" ARE TEMPORARY. Take a few minutes to figure out how long you've been feeling bad. Chances are you'll realize that your mood has only lasted a couple of days.

• STOP BAD HABITS. Alcohol or other mood-altering substances won't help you feel better in the long run; they'll only mask your bad mood temporarily or encourage your pain to surface in unexpected ways. Also, consider eliminating sugar from your diet for at least a month—it's known to have a depressive effect on the body.

• TAKE NUTRITIONAL SUPPLEMENTS. Experts suggest that nutritional supplements such as vitamin E, calcium, or evening primrose oil might reduce symptoms of depression. St. John's wort is an herb that works as an antidepressant with few side effects, provided you wait two to four weeks for it to take effect. B vitamins may help relieve stress.

• EXERCISE. Aerobic exercise—running, walking, swimming, and cycling—stimulates the endorphins of the brain, creating a natural peace and calm.

• THINK POSITIVE THOUGHTS. Self-talk is one of the most powerful therapies for treating depression. Change your thoughts to focus on the positive. Repeating a positive affirmation to music is a powerful way to penetrate the subconscious. This creation of a healing energy and vibration is called a mantra. Here's one to try: There is only one power in this universe, God, and in God I put my trust.

- KEEP A JOURNAL. Take a half hour each day to write what you've been feeling. Don't censor yourself, just write. Purging the negative feelings will be a sweet relief.

- PAMPER YOURSELF. Take a warm, fragrant, candlelit bath. Drink some soothing chamomile tea.

- BREATHE. Stand or sit up straight and pull air in through your nose down to your abdomen. Feel your stomach area fill with air. Hold it in for a second, then exhale through pursed lips. Visualize yourself just pushing that negativity inside you to where it belongs —out. As you breathe, think, I breathe out fear and breathe in light and love.

Sometimes a bad mood is a reaction to external events—a fight with your partner, the kids working your nerves, or something as small as having a bad hair day. But if something good happens—a phone call from an old friend, a raise at work, you win the lottery—that funk would disappear pretty fast, wouldn't it? But let's say that your mood persists for longer than two weeks, and nothing you do helps you to shake it off. You get praise at work or assurance from your mate, but you still feel your life could be better. This is more serious; you may be suffering from a clinical depression and should get some help.

TONI MORRISON

I WENT INTO A DEEP DEPRESSION AFTER THE FIRE IN MY HOME. I WAS PREPARED TO STAY IN THAT DEPRESSION AND NOT WRITE ANYTHING. BUT THEN I REALIZED THIS WILL PASS OR IT WON'T. I HAVE NO TRICKS. THE TRICK IS TO RIDE IT OUT.

Right: Lavender is a soothing scent.
Opposite: Herbal teas and time spent alone can help to calm and renew.

THE DOWN-HOME BATH

Cedar, perhaps because of its associations with country life, old hope chests, or holiday spirits, is said to calm, comfort, and warm the spirits for a sensual, harmonious feeling. The blend of essential oils is also useful as a massage oil.

2 drops cedar
2 drops clary sage
2 drops lavender
2 drops orange
2 tablespoons canola, olive, or almond oil

Mix the oils and stir them into a warm bath. Drift off to whatever daydream springs to mind. For a variation that may stir uplifting memories of straightening or curling hair on a Saturday night, substitute four drops of bergamot for the cedar. If romance is part of the evening's plan, try vanilla, chamomile, rose, and lavender in a bath or massage oil. For the "my one last good nerve" cure, try geranium, lavender, clary sage, lemon balm, and orange. Add candlelight and soft music, then go right to bed—alone or not.

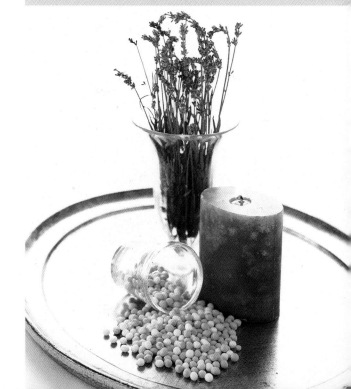

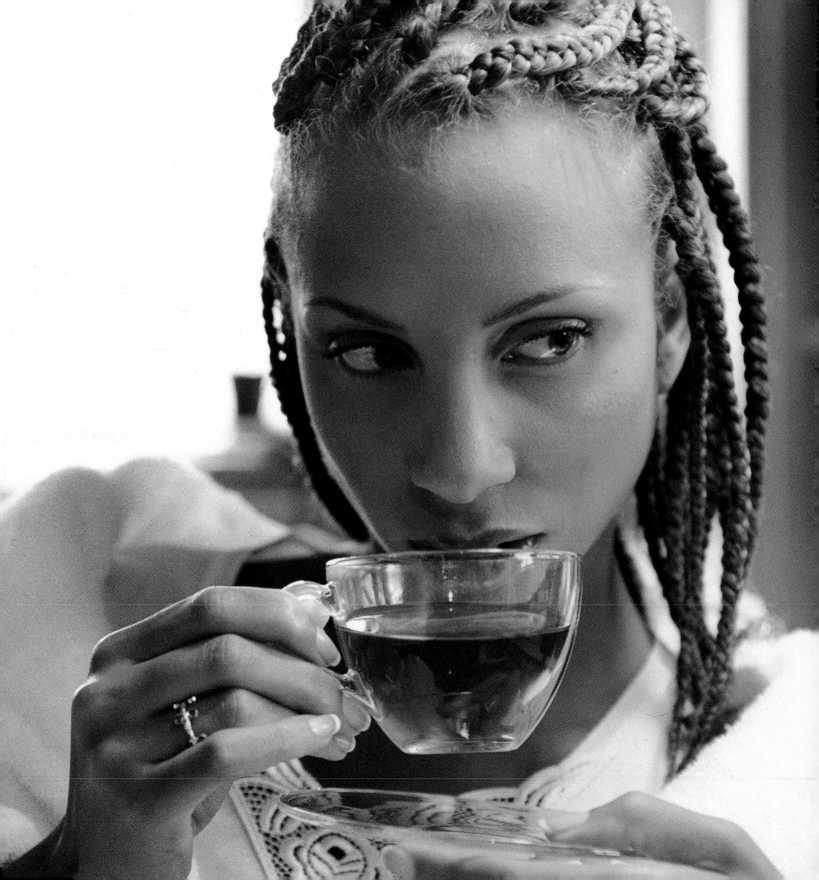

DEPRESSION

Depression can be caused by any combination of factors—biological, genetic, or psychological. It can come on gradually or suddenly, and stay with you longer than you might expect. In times of extreme stress or grief you feel depressed as a natural reaction to things you can explain, such as a death in the family. There are other times, though, when you get that sad, sinking feeling and can't explain why life is going well yet nothing can make you smile.

If you're suffering from depression, regardless of the root cause, you very likely have feelings of overwhelming sadness. You may weep uncontrollably, or you may be emotionless and numb to the world. You may sleep too much, or not at all. Your weight may balloon up, or drop dramatically. Life may not interest you.

This is not something you have brought on yourself. It doesn't mean that you're too weak to handle life, or too lazy to do something about the feelings you're having. Clinical depression is a medical illness, and it *can* be treated. If your pain outweighs your pleasure most of the time, get in touch with a mental health professional.

Mental health professionals advocate a four-prong approach to getting help. Read them over, discuss them with a friend or your spiritual advisor, and take the first step.

• GET A COMPLETE PHYSICAL EXAMINATION. This allows you to identify any medical conditions that might be affecting your mental health.

• LEARN WHAT TREATMENT OPTIONS ARE AVAILABLE TO YOU. Be aware that there are several roads you can take to feeling better—support groups, psychotherapy, medication, and others—and you must be proactive and choose the path that's right for you.

• FIND A MENTAL HEALTH SPECIALIST. They can help guide you through your specific challenges.

• PARTICIPATE IN YOUR OWN HEALING. Spend time reflecting on your life and get clarity about the things that cause you pain. Commit to ridding your life of negative people and any behaviors that aren't life supporting.

COPING WITH LOSS

The death of a loved one can trigger feelings of intense loss and can have a tremendous impact on the way you live your life. In time, however, you can expect your feelings of grief to fade enough to enable you to go on with your life. Sometimes that's difficult to do, but once you identify the source of your pain, the work toward healing begins. Going about that healing in a positive way can help you restore your sense of balance sooner rather than later.

Healing often comes in four steps: denial, bargaining, anger, and acceptance. Grief counselors help us to understand that rejecting the reality of our loss, or denial—This can't be happening to me!—is a natural first reaction to a death. You may feel that prolonging your mourning of a deceased loved one keeps his or her memory closer. You pretend to yourself that he or she hasn't really "gone on."

At some point, when you are ready, you can acknowledge the fact that your loved one's physical self is gone. Then, experts say, you may try to make a deal—with your loved one, with God, or with yourself: I'll do anything if I can just wake up in the morning and you're still here!

Eventually, you stop bargaining and confront the emotion of having been "left behind." You might be angry—with your loved one for leaving, with God for taking that person away, or with yourself for letting them go. In time, you develop a sense of acceptance and find a place of peace with the memory of your loved one.

You must allow yourself the time and space to go through the natural process of grieving. Angry? Let it out. Feel depressed? Cry it out. Need to talk it out? Call a friend.

You may feel the need to be strong and put up a good front. Cutting the grieving process short often leads to what is called "troubled mourning" and can cause you to let your grief out in other ways. Neglecting your natural need to grieve may lead to physical illness, or you may substitute some self-destructive behavior, such as excessive drinking, to help you forget your grief. It's harder for some of us to let go than for others. So you have to give yourself time to heal.

SURVIVING A LOSS

Everyone's grief is unique in its manifestation and duration, but experts offer these tips for surviving the loss.

CONSULT THE SPIRIT. Now is the time to seek spiritual guidance to help understand human passages and the cycles of life. Joining a spiritual community also provides relationships that aid healing.

STUDY THE SUBJECT. Read books on grieving to learn about loss and come to terms with it. Find sources and support groups on the Internet or through hospitals, therapists, and librarians.

TALK, TALK, TALK. Frequent chats with a trusted friend, lover, or therapist can help to relieve tensions, offer perspective, and maintain crucial human contact. Ask someone to be a telephone buddy.

CONSIDER THERAPY. Join a short-term bereavement group. Feelings of hopelessness or guilt are common, but these feelings must be dealt with.

ALLOW TIME TO HEAL. The grief process can't be rushed; mourning is a normal process, not a moral failing. Use all your bereavement leave and take an occasional day off later.

TAKE CARE OF YOU. Pamper yourself, get out, buy something to cuddle with, and stay involved in life. Listen to soothing music, but avoid painful movies, television, or articles for now.

PAY ATTENTION TO YOUR DREAMS. They can offer important clues to your feelings and your relationship with the deceased.

HONOR YOUR LOST ONE. Establish traditions that honor the deceased and cherish mementos. Set up a memorial, perhaps just by planting a tree or through a scholarship.

Loss can take on many faces, from grieving about a divorce or separation, to mourning the loss of your ability to bear children, to losing your job. Allow yourself time to explore all of your feelings. Without this freedom, you might find yourself in a constant state of agitation. You don't have to swallow the pain. By letting it out you purge it, and make way for the good times again.

Below: A cherished moment. *Opposite:* A strong relationship takes two whole and healthy people.

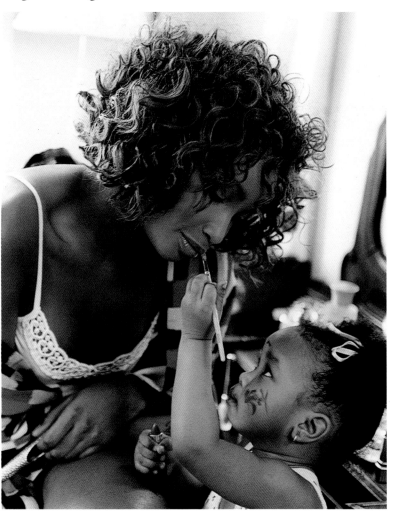

RELATIONSHIPS

Relationships provide us with the opportunity to share ourselves with others on many levels, by living in physical, emotional, intellectual, and spiritual closeness with others. We all have a need or desire for intimacy, and much of our energy is placed in seeking, building, and nurturing our relationships.

Know Your Family, Know Yourself

Most of us begin life with one of the most defining relationships we are ever likely to have—that of parent and child. Brothers and sisters might be added to create the core unit that helps to form our earliest view of the world—the family. In the beginning, you are the "child" part of that equation; later, you might become a parent. The nature of family ties are likely to influence other relationships in your life. Your family patterns affect you— by building your character, influencing your self-image, shaping your belief systems, and giving you your first experience with loving and being loved.

Reaching that understanding means taking a long, thoughtful look at how relationships have played out in our families. Draw an emotional family tree to explore the ways in which your parents, siblings, and extended family have affected your life. You might be surprised to discover just how these relationships deter-

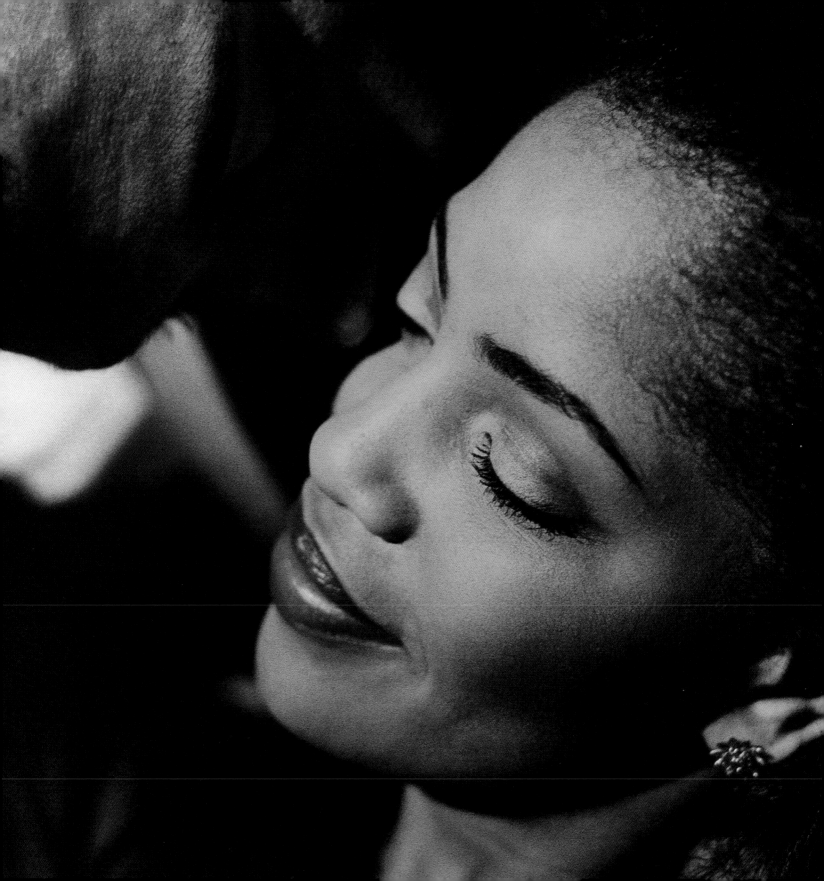

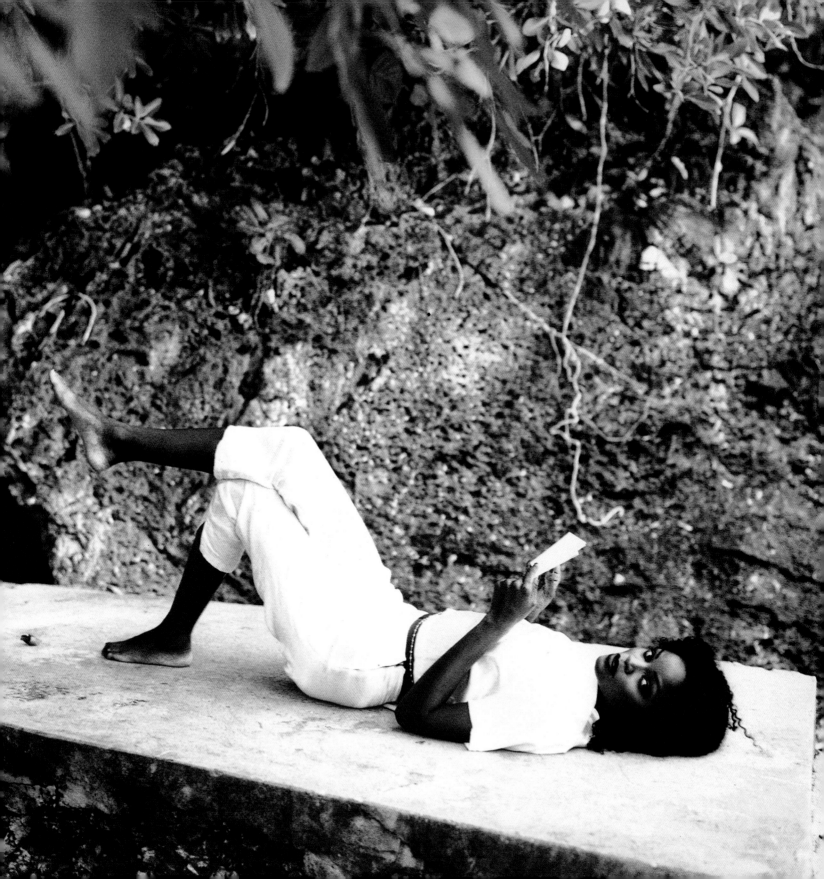

mine the way in which you interact with others in your larger world.

Make Friends with Yourself

Love makes the world go round. We all want the people in our lives to value, respect, and love us. Yet true intimacy comes from your own sense of knowing yourself. It's important to feel good about yourself and your accomplishments, for your own peace.

Many times we define ourselves in relation to the people in our lives. You might be somebody's mother, wife, daughter, or friend. Remember to cherish yourself as a complete human being, loved and honored for your beauty, inside and out. Take time to make friends with yourself.

• PRAISE YOUR PHYSICAL SELF. Make it a ritual to get in front of the mirror every morning and give thanks for the gift of your body, a magnificent one that takes you wherever you want to go. Tell yourself you're an absolutely blessed woman. And treat yourself like one.

• GIVE PRAISES TO THE UNFAILING SPIRIT INSIDE OF YOU. Take time to meditate or read inspirational passages that remind you that you are more than you seem, more than meets the eye. Feel grateful that you are always in God's care.

• LEARN TO TRUST YOUR OWN THOUGHTS AND DECISIONS. Hold on to what you believe in. Extend this practice into more and more parts of your life. Little decisions that

don't seem like much today can build into bigger, even life-altering changes tomorrow. You'll learn that you are well equipped to handle whatever life throws your way.

• MAKE FRIENDS WITH YOUR PARTNER. Take as much time to learn about your own wants, needs, and feelings as you do your partner's. A healthy partnership is made up of two whole and growing people, not halves hoping to be whole. If you are in a relationship:

• Know each other well before committing to a partnership.

• Be realistic about your expectations of your partner.

• Be willing to keep your commitment.

• Be willing to make your partnership your primary relationship.

• Maintain a sense of humor.

• Communicate with each other.

If Things Fall Apart

Despite our best efforts, sometimes relationships just don't work. Like the song says, you've got to know when to hold 'em, know when to fold 'em. If you've tried and are now convinced that it's time to part company, try to find some life lessons in leaving. You will end up in a better place.

• BE HONEST ABOUT THE RELATIONSHIP. Don't tear your ex down to build yourself back up. Your recovery from the pain of separation depends in part on how willing you are to be honest about the other person, about

Opposite: Take time to relax and renew.

yourself, and about the experience you've both been through.

• DON'T FIX BLAME. You feel hurt, or resentful, but how does it help to blame your exiting or ex-partner? Blame is a waste of your time and energy.

• DON'T BLAME YOURSELF. It's not your fault, either.

• FIGHT THOSE VINDICTIVE FEELINGS. You have more positive things to do with your time than "get even."

ADDICTIONS

Addictions ruin lives. We can become addicted to just about anything—substances, people, or activities like gambling or shopping—and these things can send our lives reeling out of control. Some of us look for solace in a drink, a pill, a pipe, or a joint. Others light up a cigarette, hoping to soothe jangled nerves, only to find years later that kicking the habit isn't so easy.

Naturally, not everyone who drinks or smokes is addicted. So how do you know if you have a problem? Well, you are probably okay if: you can have a drink without it having negative effects in your life; you drink in moderation and know when to stop; alcohol is a complement to your activities, not the primary focus of what you do.

You have a problem with substance abuse if: you frequently get into trouble with family, friends, significant others, and the law as a result of your excesses; you drink or use drugs to escape your worries or troubles; you become unreasonably angry or aggressive; your tolerance level has increased exponentially, meaning that you have to drink or use more and more often to get the same results; you suffer blackouts or can't remember parts of the night before; you feel anxious, have trouble sleeping, and feel lethargic and depressed; you engage in unsafe sex while intoxicated; you've lost your job; your finances and home are in complete disarray.

Once you surrender power over your life to a potentially harmful outside force, you lose your self-control. This is an addiction.

What can you do about addictions? Get help! Whatever your addiction is, there is a treatment program that can help you to break the chains and restore your control over your own life. Recovery programs such as Alcoholics Anonymous and Gamblers Anonymous encourage you to change your self-destructive behavior and begin to develop healthy ways of handling your troubled feelings.

If you are fortunate enough to have learned how to cope with life's challenges early enough in life to avoid addiction, but know (or suspect) that others close to you have not been so fortunate, it's important to help them. Support drug prevention programs in our schools, antismoking legislation, and drug-treatment programs.

EATING DISORDERS

Not so long ago, eating way too much or way too little was not given much "weight" in our community. Now we know overeating, as well as anorexia and bulimia, are acknowledged health risks and must be openly discussed. We all know at least one sister, maybe even ourselves, who has turned to or away from food in unhealthy ways and for unhealthy reasons.

Over 50 percent of Black women are overweight. Much of the social life in the Black community has revolved around the kitchen, and the preparation and consumption of generous servings of down-home cooking. But compulsive eating habits or overeating often signal emotional issues that require more than casual attention. In the extreme, it is not unlike those obsessions we discussed in the section on addiction; instead of cocaine or alcohol, the abused substance is food.

Food can be abused through undereating as well. Increasing numbers of young sisters are becoming more obsessed with weight and engaging in damaging practices intended to control weight gain. Though less prevalent, yet no less life threatening than obesity, anorexia (a psychological disturbance that ordinarily involves some combination of excessive dieting, strenuous exercise, and abuse of diuretics and laxatives) and bulimia (the cycle of bingeing and self-induced vomiting) are growing concerns in our community.

We need to understand why some of us become compulsive overeaters while others binge and purge. If you think you've got problems with food, grab a pen and a notebook and write out your feelings. What leads to your overeating? Are you angry? Anxious? Lonely? Are you looking for reassurance from your mate? Express your feelings rather than build a wall around yourself with weight or by starving yourself. Ask for what you need. Repeat this affirmation to yourself: *I deserve love and support, and to have a healthy body.* If you need extra help, check out Overeaters Anonymous, a twelve-step program for those with similar struggles.

MONEY PROBLEMS

Lots of us consider ourselves to be very responsible and levelheaded about money matters. We generally make our own day-to-day money management decisions, resist the temptation to incur debt for frivolous reasons, and have some sense of the importance of financial planning. We are able to manage our daily affairs and meet our bills, but have no cushion against hard times. Depending on how we handle them, money-related problems can lead to dangerous levels of stress, anxiety, and emotional crisis.

As a group we sisters have more money than we've ever had before. Even so, nearly half of the Black population is still classified as poor or near poor. Our average annual income is 40 percent less than that of white Americans, yet we usually have at least as much debt as others. Older Black women are retiring without adequate savings, our young sisters and brothers are being denied educational opportunities because of attacks on affirmative action programs and rising college costs, and many more of us are now struggling to make ends meet. We have good reason to be concerned.

Take time to figure out how you can create financial stability. Plan for your future and the future of those who depend on you. Seek professional advice about investing and develop a plan to monitor your investments. Plan ahead for important expenses—such as purchasing a home, educating your children, or yourself. Review your retirement plan and take an active role in making it work to your maximum advantage. Good planning beats worrying every time. It can help to relieve the tension in your pocketbook and put your mind at ease.

Even the most careful planner can have deep-seated and long-lasting periods when they dig themselves into a debtor's hole. You might buy things you don't need or can't afford for reasons that you only partially understand, and can't see how you'll ever get in the clear again. You stop answering the phone for fear that a creditor is on the other end of the line. You're afraid to collect the mail, knowing that the bills will just keep on coming. You're irritable, nervous, and angry with yourself for allowing things to get so far out of control. What can you do?

Get help in relieving yourself of this debt through advice available from books on money management, professional financial advisers, debt relief, and consumer counseling services. Here are some practical suggestions.

• TRACK YOUR SPENDING. For two weeks, keep a small notebook solely for this purpose. Jotting down what you buy, when, and why you buy it can help you to develop a better understanding of your spending habits.

• PAY YOUR BILLS. Work out payment schedules with your creditors and stick to them. Sell everything you don't really need and apply the money to your bills. Consider cutting up most of your credit cards.

• CONTROL YOUR FUTURE SPENDING. Before you spend, stop and ask yourself, "Is this something I really need?" Most likely, you'll find that while you may want something, you don't necessarily need it.

• BREAK YOUR SPENDING HABITS. Think about why you handle money the way you do. Break free of any damaging habits.

When we lose control over parts of our lives, we tend to blame ourselves or others and feel ashamed or guilty. This doesn't help. Beating yourself up can actually prevent you from taking the strong, positive action needed to straighten out your finances and get rid of that terrible anxiety that accompanies being broke. No matter what your financial picture, as long as you're taking positive action, the glass will always be half-full instead of half-empty.

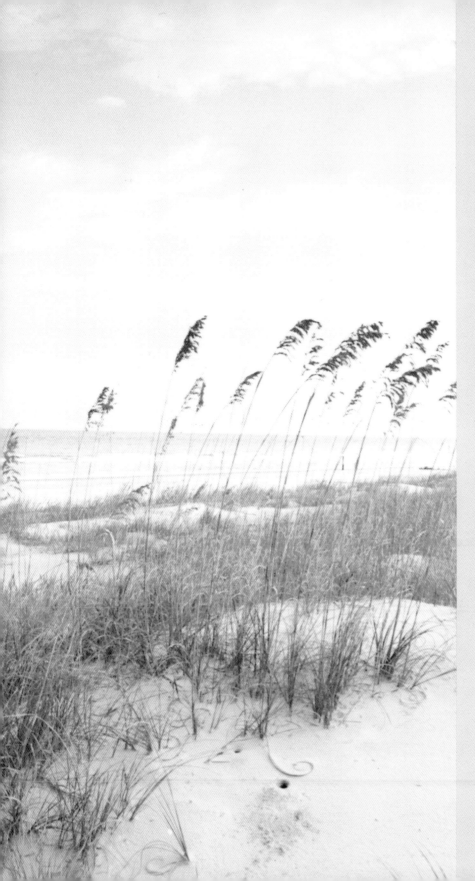

SAVE NOW!

PAY YOURSELF FIRST. Put away money before you collect it if possible, through automatic wage deductions for a credit union, savings bonds, company stock programs, or a money market fund. If your employer doesn't offer those, write a check or set up automatic transfer from checking to savings. Start now, even if you can barely spare $1 each payday, then strive for $10 a payday. If you are fortunate to start with $10 or $100 or $1,000, the principle is the same: Increase the portion you save as long as you can handle it.

BUILD A CUSHION. Work toward an emergency fund to cover three to six months' living costs. (If you are a couple, make it three to six times combined salaries and keep some assets jointly and some in each name.) Keep it in safe, liquid assets, like a money market fund, and tap into it only in dire circumstances.

INVEST FOR COMFORT. Try a three-pronged approach: Know where you are, know where you would like to be in five to ten years, and know how to get there (including what you can afford to lose). Options include tax-deferred annuities, 401(K) retirement funds, pension plans, and stock plans, all of which may be matched by employers. Do research on certificates of deposit, stocks, money markets, treasury bills, and bonds.

Opposite: Tranquil places.

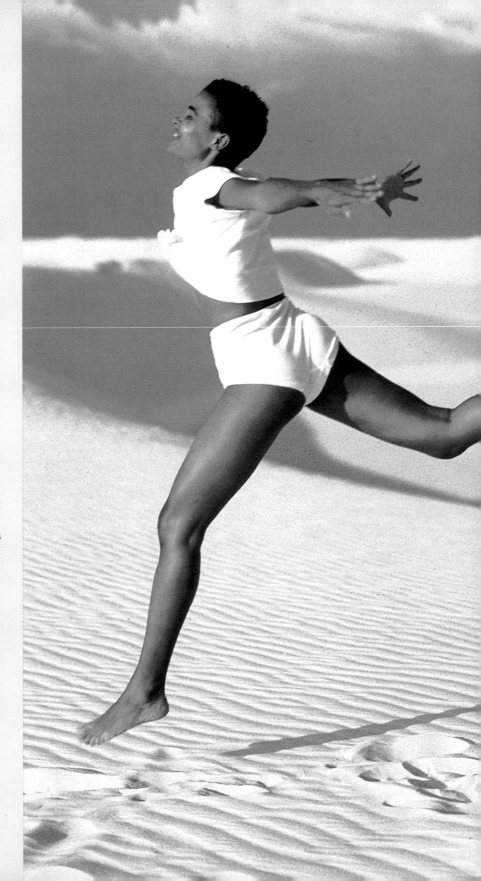

MAJOR MOOD SWINGS

Some of us have mood cycles that swing from terrible lows to phenomenal highs. This condition is called bipolar or manic-depressive disorder and affects about one in every hundred people. This particular form of depression may be due to heredity, a neurological chemical imbalance, or the result of a head injury or some other medical condition. Take the time to look at the following symptoms for mania. Check those that sound like what you're going through.

If in addition to depression, you have five or more of these manic symptoms all day, almost every day for at least two weeks, you may be undergoing a bout of serious manic depression and need to get in touch with your doctor or a mental health professional.

SIGNS OF MANIC DEPRESSION
- Feeling unusually "high," or irritable
- Requiring much less sleep
- Having swiftly changing feelings of greatness and low self-worth
- Feeling more talkative than usual, and feel pressured to talk
- Having racing thoughts and difficulty focusing
- Feeling easily distracted
- Doing things that feel good but have bad effects
- Needing to be constantly active

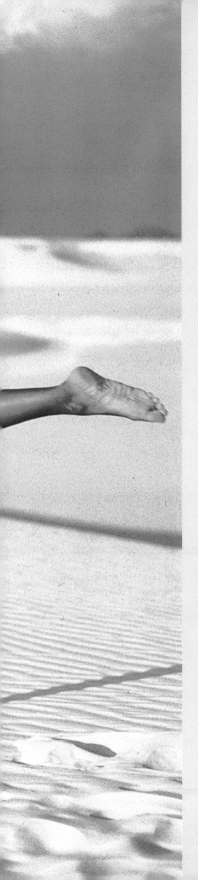

FINDING THE RIGHT THERAPIST

Many of us balk at the notion of seeking professional help with our personal problems. Just the thought of baring our souls and exposing our weaknesses to a total stranger is difficult to entertain. But our old perceptions of psychotherapy and its value, specifically to Black women, are changing. We are no longer as concerned with being viewed as crazy or "mental," and we are more receptive to the coping skills a good mental health practitioner can help us to develop—whether in crisis intervention or managing the stress and tension of everyday life. We can also look to our friends, family, and partners for advice and comfort, and generally find it.

Yet, there are times in our lives when those closest to us can't give us the kind of help we need. It may even be that they're part of the problem, so they can't be part of the solution. A therapist doesn't have the emotional attachment to you that your friends and family have, and can see your problems more objectively. Searching out a therapist can be a gift that you give yourself.

Finding the right therapist for you, however, can be an intimidating prospect. Here are a few compass points to get you started in the right direction.

TRY TO PINPOINT YOUR PROBLEM. Take your time and think about the symptoms causing you concern or unhappiness. The self-assessment questions at the beginning of the chapter may help. You should discuss these symptoms with your therapist.

ASK AROUND. Get referrals from your physician, a friend who's undergone therapy, or organizations such as the Association of Black Psychologists, Black Psychiatrists of America, the National Association of Black Social Workers, or the National Black Women's Health Project.

DO SOME RESEARCH. There are several kinds of mental health professionals with somewhat different areas of specialization. A *psychiatrist* is a medical doctor who specializes in the diagnosis and treatment of mental or psychiatric disorders. A *clinical/counseling psychologist* holds a doctorate in psychology and is trained in counseling, psychotherapy, and psychological testing. A *social worker* generally has a master's degree in social work and is trained in counseling. A *psychiatric nurse specialist* is a registered nurse with a master's degree in psychiatric nursing and is trained to treat mental or psychiatric disorders.

INTERVIEW SEVERAL THERAPISTS. Most therapists will encourage you to meet with them to share information before making a decision to begin treatment. You should be comfortable enough with the person you select to establish the bond of trust you will need for successful therapy. You may be most comfortable with a Black therapist, or a woman, or a Black woman.

ASK QUESTIONS. You will want information about educational preparation, experience, approach to therapy, attitude toward medication, cost, and terms. You have the right to ask, and most professionals will encourage your questions.

BE WILLING TO CHANGE THERAPISTS IF NECESSARY. It's important that you feel satisfied with your treatment and the professional you have selected to help guide you back to emotional health. If that's not happening, try someone new.

THE MAKEOVERS

When our bodies are worn out and run down, many times all it takes is a few days of bed rest and we're up and out again. But what do we do when our mind is tired? Sometimes we are down so long we don't know which way is up. How do we climb out of that rut we're in? *Essence* helped two sisters explore their problems with professionally trained therapists.

Lynn

Everything had been running smoothly in Lynn's life. Yet after a rapid-fire string of misfortunes—the breakup with a boyfriend, two successive setbacks at her job, and the poor health of her aging mother—Lynn was asking, "What's wrong with me?" *Essence* introduced her to Dr. Beatrice Brown, a holistic psychologist in Mount Vernon, New York, to help her examine her life and uncover the hows and whys of her back-to-back challenges.

At their first session together, Lynn explained to Dr. Brown that because she knew her mother's sickness was out of her hands and that she took responsibility for her work-related stresses, she was most concerned about her relationships and the way she communicated with people. More specifically, she wanted to know why she continually gravitated toward non-rewarding relationships with men.

Dr. Brown knew that many times the reasons our adult lives are the way they are grow from seeds sown in childhood, so she guided Lynn back to her early years of development to examine unresolved childhood issues. In order to open herself to a deeper level of consciousness, Dr. Brown had Lynn lie down on a couch to relax as she filled the air with aromatic scents and lit candles to promote relaxation. With her mind calm and reflective, Dr. Brown asked Lynn to recall the most devastating moment of her childhood.

Lynn responded by speaking about her father. During her childhood, her father was either "emotionally unavailable" or physically absent from her life. Dr. Brown suggested that this gap in her life left Lynn constantly seeking a male role model to fill that vacancy. Dr. Brown also indicated that without the bonds made in a father-daughter relationship, Lynn might have developed an insecurity about interacting with men in general, so that the distance and disassociation she felt from her father's absence spilled over and prevented her from establishing an emotional connection with men in romantic relationships as she grew older.

Over another face-to-face session and a phone conversation with Dr. Brown, Lynn examined the pattern of nonrewarding relationships in her life, and began to see that she

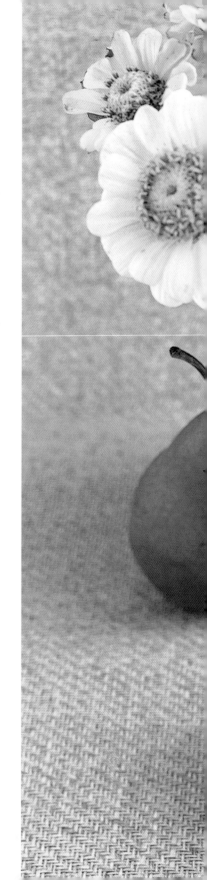

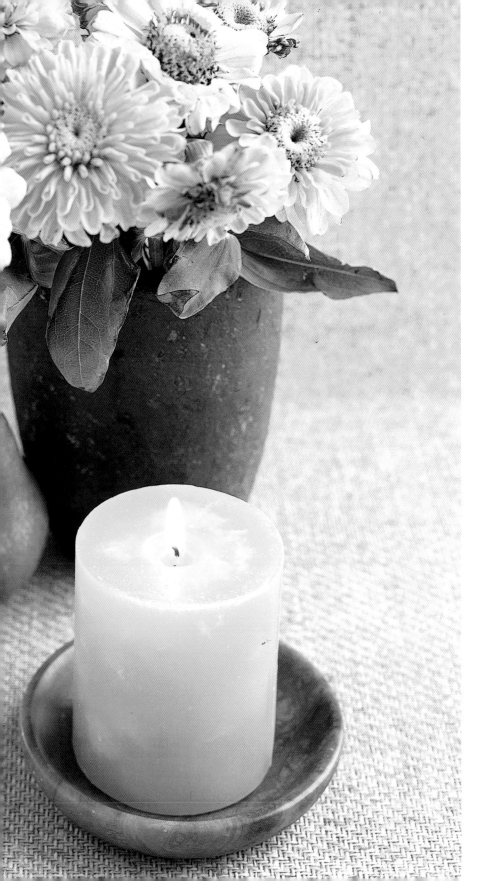

had an active role in the outcome of those relationships. Her fear of abandonment and rejection picked up in childhood had developed into a general mistrust, so that even as she enjoyed the beginning stages of dating, she always ended up pulling back emotionally until a breakup was unavoidable. Dr. Brown reassured her that casual dating is perfectly normal, but she also told Lynn that as we grow older we feel a stronger need to connect with someone on a higher level. It was probably this lack of gratification that had been distressing Lynn so much.

Even though short-term therapy isn't a quick-fix solution to a problem, Lynn knew that she could use Dr. Brown's advice and perspective to gain insight and work toward more fruitful relationships in the future.

Imani

Imani's life had been blessed with a stable circle of nurturing family members and friends, then suddenly she suffered the devastating death of her mother and her world was turned upside down. Imani's mother had been her heart, and without that presence in her life she felt lost. Dr. Linda Anderson, a New York City–based clinical psychologist, guided Imani through her grief and set her on a path toward healing herself.

Dr. Anderson said that Imani was in a "reactive depression"—a response to one of the most significant losses anyone can face in her

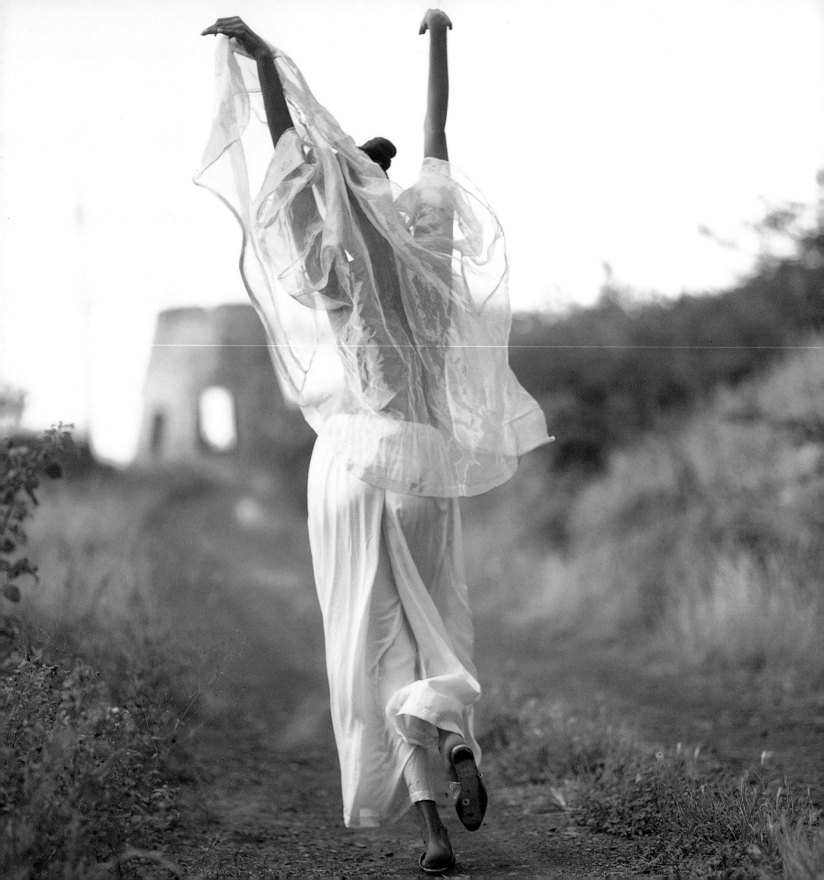

lifetime. This associated pain can be even more acute among African-American women, Dr. Anderson said, where mother-daughter bonds are often especially strong; many of the essential life lessons learned during a sister's psychological development come from the relationship with her mother. Imani's mother embodied this strong, giving, highly evolved, and spiritual type of woman we all hope to be.

Most of Dr. Anderson's work with Imani centered on increasing her self-awareness and coping strategies, restoring her zest for life and reestablishing her connection to the loved ones around her. One of the simplest ways to do this, Dr. Anderson suggested, was for Imani to do a self-care "check in" with herself at various points during the day. Like a lot of sisters, Imani had a high-pressure job, and that made it even more important for her to stop and ask herself, "How am I doing?" and "What do I need to do for myself today?" This sort of self-care, along with deep breathing, creative visualization, and simple stretching, can be instrumental in processing and understanding our emotions during a period of grief or depression.

As Imani and Dr. Anderson explored other avenues of relational self-therapy, Dr. Anderson noted that while Imani was in the midst of grieving, she was also in an intense period of personal change. As a young woman in her early twenties, Imani was experiencing the process of "individuation"—a time in which she was becoming fully responsible for taking care of herself. Although it was painfully difficult not to have her mother's guidance as she approached independent adulthood, Dr. Anderson helped Imani begin to understand her mother's passing better and to take all those positive qualities Imani remembered her for and integrate them into her own life. In the future, this process will ultimately bear fruit as Imani considers becoming the sort of partner, mother, and friend to others that her mother had been.

Lastly, it was important for Imani to remain in touch with her feelings as she moved through her loss. Wearing a mask that said "everything is fine" would only serve to suppress her true emotions, forcing them below the surface until they blew up and backfired in unexpected ways. Dr. Anderson told her that on average it takes a person's psyche three years to heal from the sort of pain she was going through, so being honest and open about how she felt was important to putting her grief into a framework she could understand and live with.

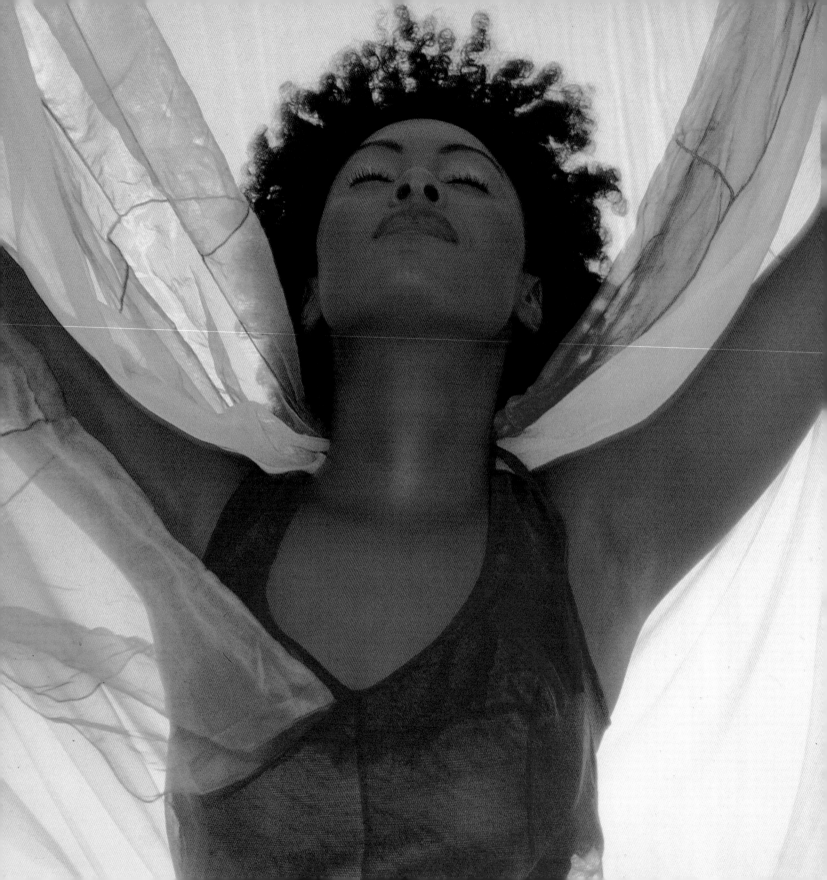

6 SPIRITUAL POWER

WHO DO YOU THINK YOU ARE? When we were kids, that question may have come as a schoolyard taunt. But as adults, this provocative question is well worth asking. Consider it: If someone were to strip away all that you know to be you—your name, your personality, even your body—what would remain? In a word, spirit.

That's easy to forget in our world, where we spend almost every waking moment dealing with someone or something outside of ourselves. When things are going well, we may think, "Hey, check me out!" But when we fall short of our goals, or a romance fizzles, or a loved one passes on, we see what we're really made of. It's during those times that we do our most profound soul-searching. If we're really serious about upping our game, however, we don't wait until we've

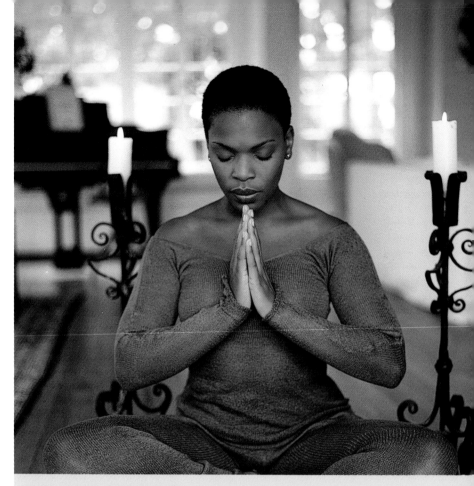

fallen into a funk to tap our soul power, we draw on it every day. This sparkling treasure at the core of each of us is our greatest asset.

Many of us got a sense of the value of spirituality as youngsters. Our parents or another God-loving relative would gather us all up for church every weekend. To them, it was paramount that we got religion. That meant a pastor, a congregation, special rituals, and a path to God—outlined in the Bible or some other sacred text—that spelled out all the dos and don'ts of life.

It was in the church that we first let our little lights shine. It was where we initially felt a sense of community. And where we learned, from the weekly announcement listing the sick and the infirm, that it was our duty to look after one another. Most important, our early introduction to faith showed us that we are far more than we seem, part, in fact, of the force that we call God. Whether we are Christian, Muslim, Buddhist, or Yoruba, our religion is a way of getting to know that force at work—an all-knowing, all-powerful Spirit that is greater than all of us at our greatest.

Spirituality is about the inner work. We simply need to be still and listen, and then allow the Holy Spirit, by whatever name, to place us on the right track. When we develop this deep, personal relationship with God, we enjoy a peace and balance in our lives— even when the world around us is spinning out of control.

SELF-ASSESSMENT

- Do you understand the difference between religion and spirituality?
- Do you have a spiritual belief system that works for you?
- Do you take time each day to pray or meditate?
- Do you have faith?
- Are you loving toward yourself? Are you open to receiving love?
- Have you let go of the past and forgiven those who have hurt you?
- Do you welcome change as a vital part of life?
- Can you see evidence of abundance in your life and feel gratitude for it?
- Do you feel inner peace?
- Do you have hope for the future?

If you answered "yes" to a majority of these questions, you are aware of the importance of spirituality in your life, and you are probably open to new ideas on how to embrace your serenity, joy, and spiritual well-being. If you answered "yes" to less than half of the questions, the best is yet to come. Look to this chapter for information on building blocks to guide and strengthen your lifelong spiritual journey.

To put it another way: If religion is the frame that supports and gives shape to our relationship with God, then spirituality might be the painting we put in the frame. We choose the colors, the texture, the images, and the shapes—hey, it's our painting.

Within this chapter are ideas for enhancing serenity, joy, and spiritual well-being. Some of them may resonate with your soul.

Spirit speaks to us in a language all its own. It whispers to us through intuition, dreams, feelings, vibrations. When we're tuned in, we move through the world happy for no particular reason. We delight in the simplest things: a child's smile, the bright face of a sunflower. When we pass a mirror, we may glance at ourselves and wink. Our inner lives and outer selves are aligned, and the payoff is a serene contentment.

When we give our spirit short shrift, however, we may experience a vague void within. Or sometimes it's an odd sadness, especially during those moments—say, following the job promotion or after we're sporting the shiny new car—when we'd think we'd be kicking up our heels with delight.

To get in touch with the state of your spirit, begin to look at the underpinnings of your life. Ask yourself the following questions as you ponder where you are within and where you'd like to be.

QUEEN LATIFAH
WHATEVER YOU WANT TO DO AND WHEREVER IT IS YOU WANT TO GO, SHOOT FOR IT. LISTEN TO THAT BIG, LOUD VOICE THAT IS INSIDE ALL OF US, GUIDING US IF WE WILL ONLY PAY ATTENTION.

SEVEN PRINCIPLES OF SPIRITUALITY

It's a given: The Creator's always got our back. Still, it's not enough to kick back and lean on "the everlasting arms"; we've got to step up and create a way of being in the world that reflects our soul. A bridge cannot exist without structural support. Our lives demand the same kind of foundation. Our personal bridge to greater spiritual awareness requires the stepping-stones of purpose, faith, love, forgiveness, gratitude, truth, and peace to carry us across to a happier, more satisfying life. This journey is long, but if we keep getting up, making a little more progress each day, we'll get there when the time is right.

Here's more about the seven principles and how to make them real in your life.

PURPOSE

You are unique. No one who lived before you or who will come after you will be exactly like you. That's because each of us was created for a mighty purpose. With all the stuff on your plate, you may not feel like a superwoman, and

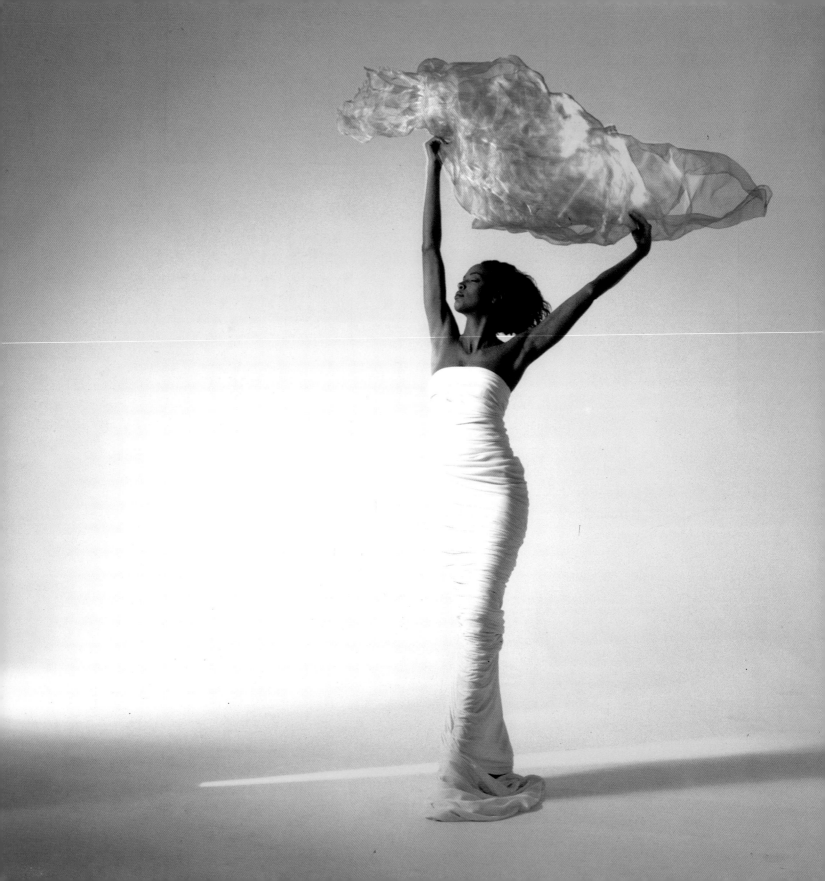

Opposite: Spiritual principles are the building blocks for your soul's growth. *Right:* Time spent at the seaside can bring inner peace for the soul.

yet you have the power to imagine something great and, bit by bit, transform that vision into reality. But that means you can't go along with just anybody's program. You have to discover the work that most nourishes *your* spirit, that sparks a glide in *your* stride—whether that means owning a business, staying home to raise a family, or learning to cut hair.

Nobody can tell you what your purpose is; it has to come from within. You can ask friends and loved ones what they see for you (and they may have some valuable insights), but ultimately you have to see it for yourself. And once you find "your calling," it's good for everyone else as well; your joy spreads to your coworkers, your community, the world around you.

To gain clarity about what God has in mind for your life, ask yourself: "What is it that I tend to do—naturally, spontaneously, voluntarily—that (a) profoundly satisfies me, (b) contributes meaningfully to others, and (c) glorifies the Creator?" Finish the statement:

"I _____."

(Be sure to choose the single most personally descriptive verb, for example, *inspire, nurture, enlighten, beautify, clarify, edify, encourage, transform, relieve, entertain, inform, motivate, serve, lead,* etc.) Don't be alarmed if it takes a few days, a few weeks, or even a few months or longer to pinpoint your divinely appointed life purpose. It's worth the wait. Once you're clear, see how the greater plan compares with your everyday life. Get on purpose. As you move through life,

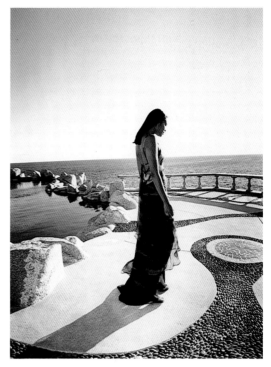

you may find that your purpose changes periodically. Be open to how the spirit moves you.

FAITH

Each of our lives is a square in God's colorful quilt. When we understand this, we know why we must pursue our destinies through thick and thin. But we need faith to get there. This trust in the power of the Creator to meet all our needs and to carry us safely across turbulent territory resides in a realm beyond reason and intellect. Faith works best when we surrender to it, remembering that things always work out—one way or another.

Sometimes, during a life-changing crisis, we

may ask how low can this go? We wonder if God has pulled a disappearing act. In the clutch of doubt and despair, it's hard to keep things in perspective. But God knows that we've got the goods to handle any situation we find ourselves in. Vague, theoretical abstractions about faith won't cut it when the heat is on. You've got to know God can deliver—no matter what.

To deepen your faith, read each morning at least one chapter of a spiritual text of your choosing. After an initial reading, stop and pray. Ask that God's abiding power be revealed to you in the passage. Read the words again, slowly, meditatively. Begin to keep a journal to summarize what the reading for the day was and how it impressed upon you God's trustworthiness. When your faith is flagging, review some of your journal entries.

LOVE

There are probably as many ways to love as there are butterflies in spring. And like butterflies who evolve from earthbound caterpillars, love uplifts us. Our minds, bodies, and spirits need love to thrive and to give us the inspiration to go on fighting the good fight. It is through the kindness we show to ourselves that we grow in self-esteem. And it is through positive relationships with others that we find the encouragement and support unity brings. Having a strong bond with God helps us con-nect with the power to transform our lives and those of people around the world.

We're charged with expanding our capacity to love on all three of these levels:

THE SELF Some of us sisters keep our hair and nails primped to a high-gloss sheen. On the outside we shine like a pile of gold coins, but not necessarily on the inside. Self-love demands that we go beyond appearances and get to work on that inside job. It's the little things, like eating well or exercising regularly, that are the real barometers on how we're doing. We have to attend to our mental health, as well. It can be enhanced in so many ways: by taking time to establish meaningful friendships, for instance, or reading nourishing books. And meditation and prayer are unparalleled in their ability to soothe the soul.

OTHERS When we feel whole, we have something to share. One of the sweetest things we can do for others is to listen to them—without judgment and without rushing in to give unasked-for advice. Loving others can mean volunteering, teaching young people, and helping our elders. What do you have to give that might brighten someone's life?

Bringing the sunshine to others is a breeze when they please us, but what about when they let us down, break our hearts, or go against our wishes? Do we stop loving them? And if we do, was it the real thing in the first place? We've got to check ourselves, and be ready to seek a higher love—one that accepts others and ourselves for

Opposite: The beauty of nature displays the wonders of our Creator.

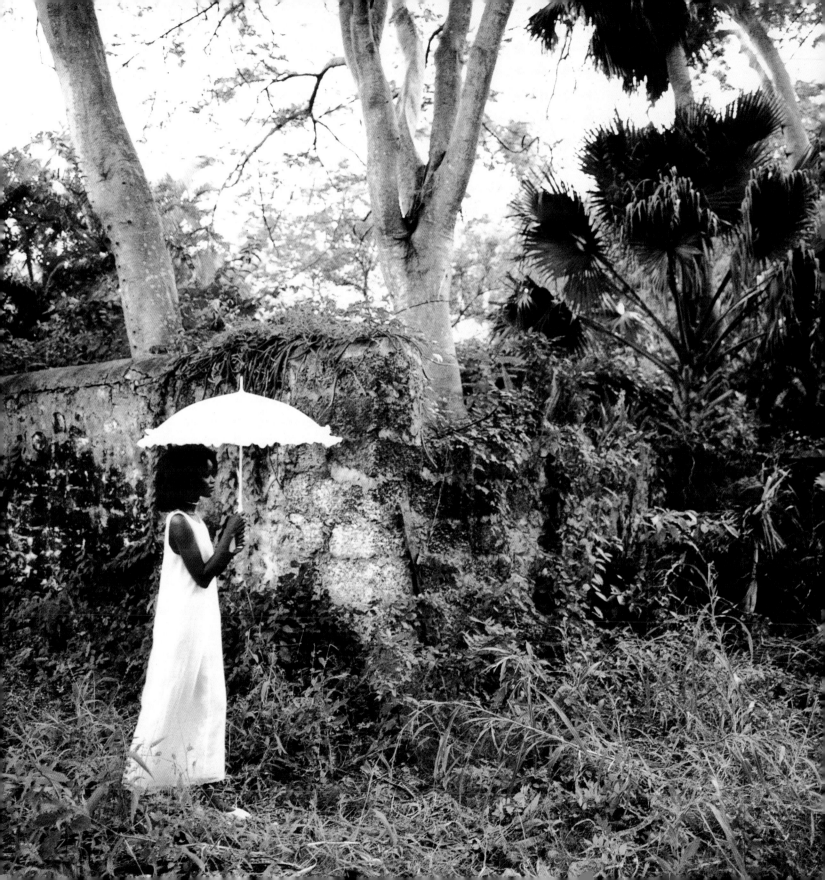

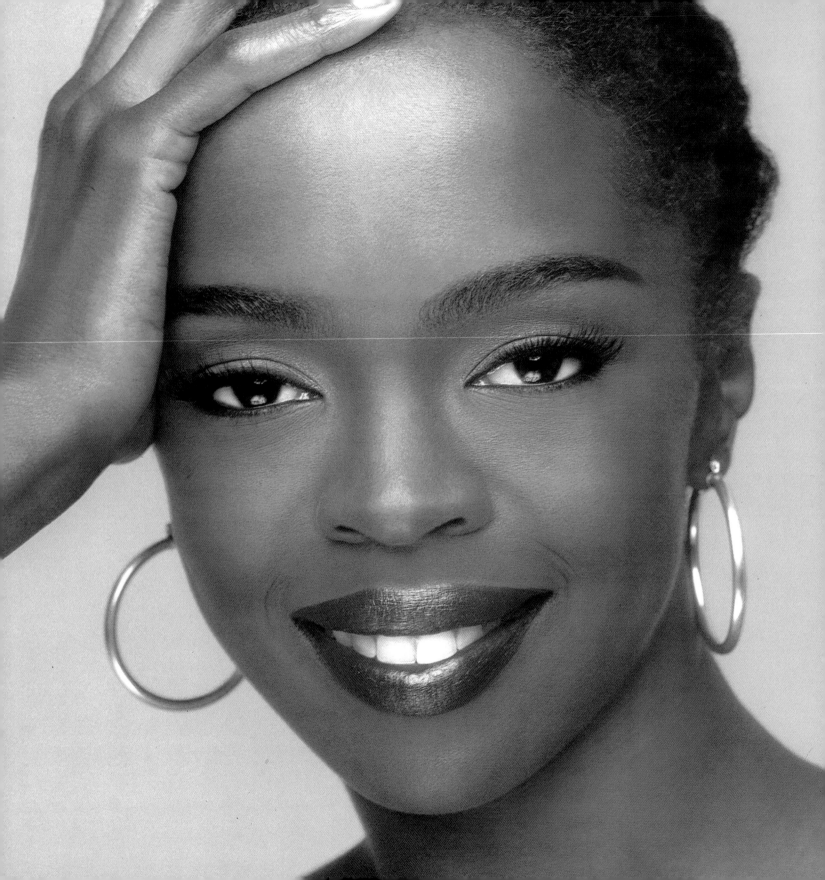

LAURYN HILL

I'VE BEEN SO SUCCESSFUL BECAUSE I RESPECT THE FACT THAT MY TALENT IS A GIFT FROM GOD. IT'S COOL IF PEOPLE GIVE US KUDOS AND ACCOLADES, BUT I KNOW WHO IS RESPONSIBLE FOR EVERYTHING I DO. ALL PRAISE SHOULD BE GIVEN TO HIM.

who we are, not for who we would have them be.

GOD We show love for the Creator by worshiping in communion with others or by reading books of Scripture or inspiration. Our devotion also means going beyond this, to spend quiet time tuned to the still, small voice of God that is always urging us on. In any way that we show love to anyone at any time, we honor the Creator.

Some of us know the power of love because someone showered us with it when we were little. Others of us know how profoundly important it is because we were denied it for too long. Identify someone in your life who, without question, best demonstrates pure, unconditional love on a daily basis. Stop and reflect on the specific ways this person exhibits these qualities to you and to others. What must you do, stop doing, or change (in your attitudes, behaviors, responses, or motives) to become more like your loving role model?

FORGIVENESS

If you want to move your life forward, you've got to recognize the power of forgiveness. For some of us, this idea is tough to swallow. We believe that if we don't keep track of all the ways people have dissed us in the past, we might fall into somebody's trick bag again. So we hold on to a wrong done to us five, ten, even twenty or more years ago. The upside—if

Opposite: Lauryn Hill.

MEDITATION

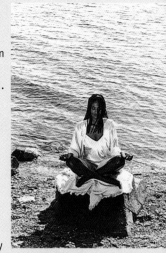

Meditation could be described as a spiritual umbilical cord that connects you to the Creator. Each time you sit down to meditate, you download a nourishing stream of soul food. At first it might be hard to sit still and peel away competing thoughts from your mind, but after you've been meditating awhile, you will find that your days feel calmer. When crises do arise, you'll trust yourself to manage them.

There are many different ways to meditate, and probably as many books on the market to tell you how. Here's one to try: Pick a quiet place where you won't be disturbed. Light a candle or your favorite incense. Sit in a chair or some place where your posture is erect—that is, with your head, neck, and back in a straight line. Take a long, slow breath, pulling air deep into the center of your body. As you inhale, imagine that your breath is a ray of light sweeping up from the base of your spinal cord to the bottom of your skull. Exhale, imagining your breath sweeping back down your spine. With your next breath, imagine it sweeping up to the crown of your head. Repeat this at least sixteen times, continuing to coordinate the breath you take in with the upward sweeping motion, and the breath you send out with the down stroke. One inhale-exhale cycle counts as one breath. Feel free to slow the speed of your breathing. When you've finished, bring your breath back to normal and sit in silence.

The full rewards of meditation are reaped when you do it consistently. Try to set aside fifteen to twenty minutes in the morning and another fifteen to twenty minutes in the evening. Your soul will open up.

there is one—is that we feel superior to the other person. The downside is that the relationship we have with that person (and sometimes with others) dies or limps along, and the wound within us never heals.

What we don't realize is that by holding on to old hurts, we block some of the love and joy that might flow into our lives if we could only let go of our resentments. To forgive, then, is to abandon the old for the new, to make room for the good and to allow life to send fresh, positive possibilities our way.

If you see some areas in your life where you could benefit from a dose of forgiveness, summon the courage to act on them. You might get the ball rolling by forgiving yourself. Were there moments in the past when you didn't quite meet a challenge or a goal you'd set for yourself? Perhaps you made a poor choice that had serious consequences. Whatever the deal was, it happened in the past and the past can't be changed. So let yourself off the hook. Instead of dragging around a sack of guilt, look for the lesson in what happened, and see every negative experience as a chance to get it right next time.

When it comes to forgiving others, it doesn't mean that you're supposed to pretend that what happened didn't happen or that it didn't matter. You might have suffered at the hands of the very people who were supposed to love you. Forgiveness sees the failure, acknowledges it for what it is, but refuses to hold the guilty parties emotionally hostage until they pay for what

A THIRTY-MINUTE VACATION

Even when your travel funds are scarce, you can still get away from it all. Slough off the pressures of the world with a "mini-vacation."

Set aside at least a half hour for yourself and hang a "do not disturb" sign outside the bathroom door. Brew yourself a soothing cup of chamomile or peppermint tea while the tub is filling with warm water. Add a couple of drops of a pleasing essential oil to the bath. Lavender is relaxing and soothing. Rose is gentle to jangled nerves and also elevates your mood. Sweet orange and other citrus oils refresh the spirits. And sandalwood chases the blues.

Light a candle or turn the dimmer switch down low. Put some slow, easy jazz on the stereo and climb into the tub—taking your tea and a good book with you.

Sip, soak, and enjoy the scent of your fragrant bath. Massage the soles of your feet if they've been demanding attention. Or perhaps just lie back and enjoy the glow.

they did. That day may never come, so why spend years waiting in pain. Give it up, turn it loose. Ultimately, the universe is fair: What you give you get. A person doesn't wound you without wounding him- or herself. If someone has caused you to suffer, that person needs your compassion and prayers to help him or her find a more loving way to be in the world.

Consider a time in your past when you did someone wrong and were desperate to receive forgiveness. Try to remember how important it was to you to be pardoned and offered a reprieve, despite how deeply you disappointed this person. Now commit to giving those who need your forgiveness the same kind of grace and mercy you craved when you were wrong. The one who wronged you is more alike than different from you.

Opposite: Jackie Lewis finds peace in yoga at her spa in Negril.

Forgiveness can prove extremely difficult to offer. If you've tried and tried and yet still find yourself stuck in that old rut, consider talking to a wise friend or a spiritual leader to help you move on to higher ground.

GRATITUDE

It'd be nice to have a fatter bankroll or the freedom to jet off to the Caribbean whenever you had the notion, but rest assured that God has given you everything you need to live in peace, joy, health, and abundance. We often take for granted the countless blessings that have been bestowed upon us. Gratitude is about being thankful for what you have *already* got.

Be thankful that you awakened this morning. Be grateful that you can dream a world and then roll up your sleeves and create it. This is what it means to be born in the image and likeness of God: You, too, have the ability to perform wonders. Feel gratitude for this great power that is in your hands. Feel gratitude that you are an earth angel, a child of God.

We miss out on the sweetness of life when we sit around, grumbling about how the glass is half empty rather than half full. If we're tapping our fingers, waiting to get glad when that high-powered job comes through, that diet whittles us down, or that man bops along, we are missing the point. It's as nutty as starving at a banquet!

But of course, as long as we're on the planet,

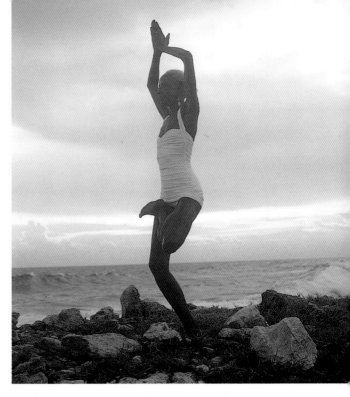

we'll long to do more and to be more. This divine discontent is a given. But don't let it suck you in.

As a demonstration of your gratitude, establish the habit of giving a "thanks offering" to God. It may be through tithing, a special ritual you devise, or by supporting a righteous cause. Perhaps you will show your praise by making a difference in another person's life, helping out with some task or need. Give simply, sincerely, and selflessly as an act of recognition for all that has been given to you.

TRUTH

One of the reasons we're driven to explore our spirituality is because we want to know the bottom line. Even as we get on purpose, grow in faith and love, work hard to forgive, and uplift ourselves and others with gratitude, we may wonder, when you break it all down, what's the point? What is life about anyway?

There's no simple answer to those questions. People have pondered them for centuries and come up with completely different conclusions. That's okay. The important thing is that we ask the question in the first place. And even as we seek answers, it helps to understand that as works-in-progress, what we come up with may only be a piece of the puzzle. So take the time to delight in the little revelations along the way, and yet don't hold on to any

AFFIRMATIONS

Before the first brick of Egypt's great pyramids was lain, someone imagined them there. All great things begin with an idea. So when we seek important change in our lives, the magic is in knowing it can be so, rather than in dwelling on how hard it will be to achieve it. An affirmation is a positive statement about yourself that you repeat over and over, until your subconscious gets the message. By changing your belief at this level, you have the power to change your reality.

Look at an area of your life where you are most in need of transformation, whether it's your physical condition, your employment, or your relationships. For example, you might affirm, "It is my divine right to take my own direction in life and to succeed. Everything I touch is a success." Write your affirmation down and say it aloud to yourself several times every morning and evening. Say it throughout the day, when you think of it. This is the first brick of your pyramids.

MAYA ANGELOU
I ENCOURAGE YOUNG BLACK WOMEN IN THE CORPORATE OFFICES, IN THE HOSPITALS, IN THE RESTAURANTS AS WAITRESSES, AT HOME AS HOMEMAKERS, TO PLAN ONE HOUR A WEEK TO GIVE TO SOMEBODY— TO AN OLD FOLKS' HOME, AN ORPHANAGE. JUST GET OFF YOUR BEHIND AND GIVE. YOU'LL BE AMAZED. YOU GET BACK MORE THAN YOU GIVE. BUT GIVE ONLY WITH THE INTENT OF GIVING.

conclusions too tightly. The process of evolving is more important than how it all turns out. Enjoy the process of allowing your life to unfold spiritually. It's truly divine!

When we see a picture of ourselves that we like, we may peek at it again and again, quietly satisfied. But when we see an unflattering image of ourselves—say, one that emphasizes those pounds we've picked up or the dental work we've been meaning to have done—it can be hard to take. Yet the feedback can be the push we need to make needed change.

Summon the courage to examine the full truth of who you are. With a pen and paper, make a list of those traits that you'd prefer no one see. Maybe you have a tendency to "read" people too quickly, or perhaps you have an intense need to control everybody and everything. When you've written the traits down, across from them put the emotion you think may be underlying the behavior. Stay conscious of the times when you revert to your unpleasant ways as you go through the week.

As we become honest about those aspects of ourselves that we find hard to accept, we make it possible to change them. And as we move away from the destructive ways of being to more positive ones, we reflect the true spirit of the Creator.

Two time-tested methods to get closer to the truth of your divine nature are prayer and meditation. They go hand in hand, and you can practice them any time and any place:

kneeling in a house of worship, lying under a tree, or even standing in line at the post office. You can do it alone, with a partner, or, if your spirit is strong enough, in the middle of a crowded room.

Some say prayer is the conduit through which the riches of heaven are brought down to earth. It is the act of prayer itself, whatever form it takes, that makes us feel God's presence most intently. We can tap the traditional prayers— the ones we learned at our mama's knees. Or we can find our own words, or use none at all. God listens to our hearts, not our words, and is happy to hear from us no matter what time we call.

In recent years, science has stepped up its study of the link between prayer and healing, but we don't need to wait for the results: We all know stories about prayer reversing a terminal illness or saving a marriage that was on its last legs, and we've seen God respond to our pleas in ways that have astounded us. If we pray on a regular basis, we know that nine times out of ten, it's not a 911 call, but more often a plea for the strength to bear up under a heavy load or to accept a situation that, despite our deepest wishes, we have no power to change. Prayer allows us to seek God's counsel, and gives us a forum to say thanks for the many miracles that have already arrived.

Consider meditation as another octave of prayer. It pulls us away from the busyness of our existence and invites us to stop, sit quietly, and focus on one thing, whether it is our

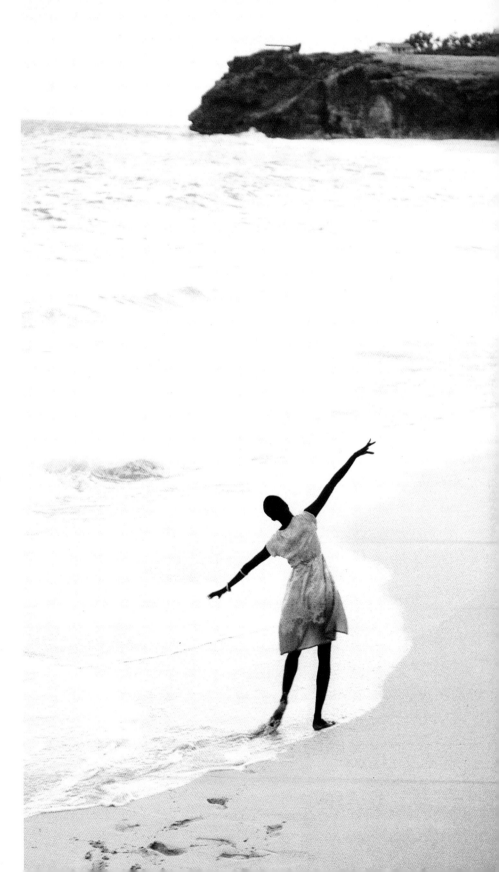

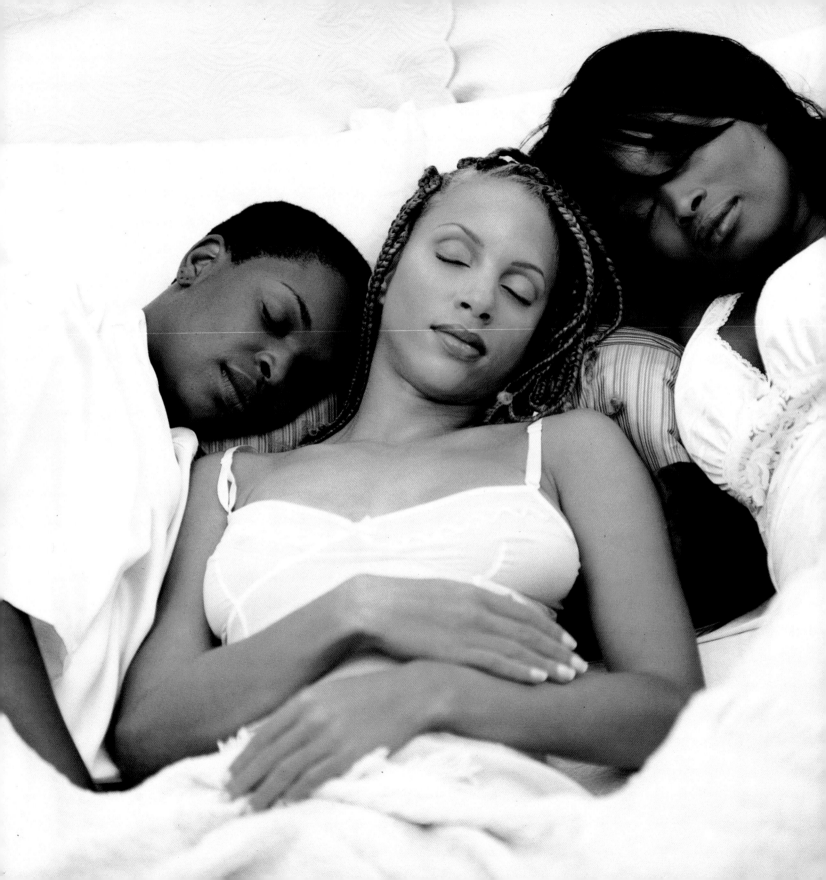

Opposite: Surround yourself with people who love and cherish you. Right: Scented linen brings comfort.

breath, a sound, or God. When we meditate, we invite our soul to come forward and grow (see page 193).

Studying the word of holy books introduces us to new ideas and insights about God. Some of us have committed ourselves to reading the Bible from cover to cover to see what it says *for ourselves,* rather than relying on the interpretation of others. Some of us read works from a variety of religious viewpoints. By studying wise words from a range of cultures, we deepen our spiritual understanding and broaden our worldview.

We richly benefit when we give ourselves the daily gift of prayer, meditation, and study.

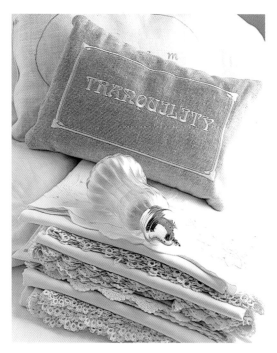

PEACE

The secret to achieving inner peace can seem elusive, especially in a culture where we're used to getting everything instantly. There is no pill, no 900 number, no magic potion that we can use to shortcut the process. We have to keep at it—sometimes proceeding in the dark —to see what contributes to our peace. It could mean ending some relationships. It may mean dropping some bad habits. As we examine our lives, we need to look at everything and ask, "Is this person, book, or experience making me more peaceful or less so?"

Once we start to reap the benefits of our spiritual quest, we have to protect it like a delicate flower—approach jealousy, envy, and other counterproductive behavior like weeds in the garden of our soul. Pluck them out. We have to surround ourselves with people who love, cherish, and support us in our quest. A chorus of like-minded folks is much stronger than a solo act.

Achieving peace is not a lofty, someday-over-the-rainbow concept. It's possible in the here and now. Establish a ritual that helps you dip into your well of peace. Make a corner of your home a place where you stop before heading out into the world. The spot could be anywhere that you can have a few moments undisturbed—your bedroom, den, or a covered outdoor patio—any place that speaks to you of tranquillity. Each day, before you head out into the world, take a few moments to stand in your

HONING INTUITION

Our elders have always encouraged us to trust "our first mind"—that is, to see how we feel about something and trust it. When you're wrestling with a problem or dilemma and you're torn, make a list of all the possible solutions. Read them over once or twice and then stop thinking about the matter altogether. Trust that the answer will come to you from God by the time you must respond. If you have a night to "sleep on it," pray that God will make the best solution.

peace corner. Hold your palms up as you imagine all the conflicts and problems gathered in them. Then, after you've given them their say, turn your palms downward and let them fall away. Imagine a divine presence filling the place where the conflict once was. You are now complete, whole; there's no room for dissension within you. As you go on your way, know that you have the power to get your needs met in the world without conflict or struggle.

When we make these seven principles the bedrock of our lives, we achieve a calming harmony and balance. We also set the stage to lead a simpler, yet more satisfying life, one that is relatively conflict-free.

Seeking Simplicity

One big block to our happiness is that too often we give our power away to pressure and panic when at any time we could reassert our authority, and hold in our hands the reins to our lives. Who doesn't feel tapped out or pulled in too many different directions? Though our list of wants may stretch on for several pages, we're better off when we concentrate on our needs, carving out time for the people who matter, paying our bills on time, getting our eyes checked. That's when our lives feel solid and secure.

We need to establish order in our immediate surroundings. If we start every morning with a mad scramble to find our keys, we've set the tone for the day and our lives will feel out of control. We must become comfortable with the word *no*. Sometimes we overcommit to others to our own detriment. We can decline anything graciously. Something simple like "I'd like to, but I won't be able to" suffices.

We need to consider our relationships—compare how we feel after spending time with a friend who's easygoing to how we feel after hanging out with one who likes to argue or complain. No contest, right? Over time, we should work to surround ourselves with positive, loving people whom we enjoy and phase out those folks who always seem to come with a side order of drama.

We're better off with people who are going in the direction in which we'd like to move. If we've made exercise a priority, perhaps finding a workout partner who will drag us out of bed for a morning run on lazy days—and for whom we can do the same—will make it easier for us both to reach our goals. Or maybe we'll make a friend, or perhaps meet a new

Opposite: Joy is a natural expression of spirituality.

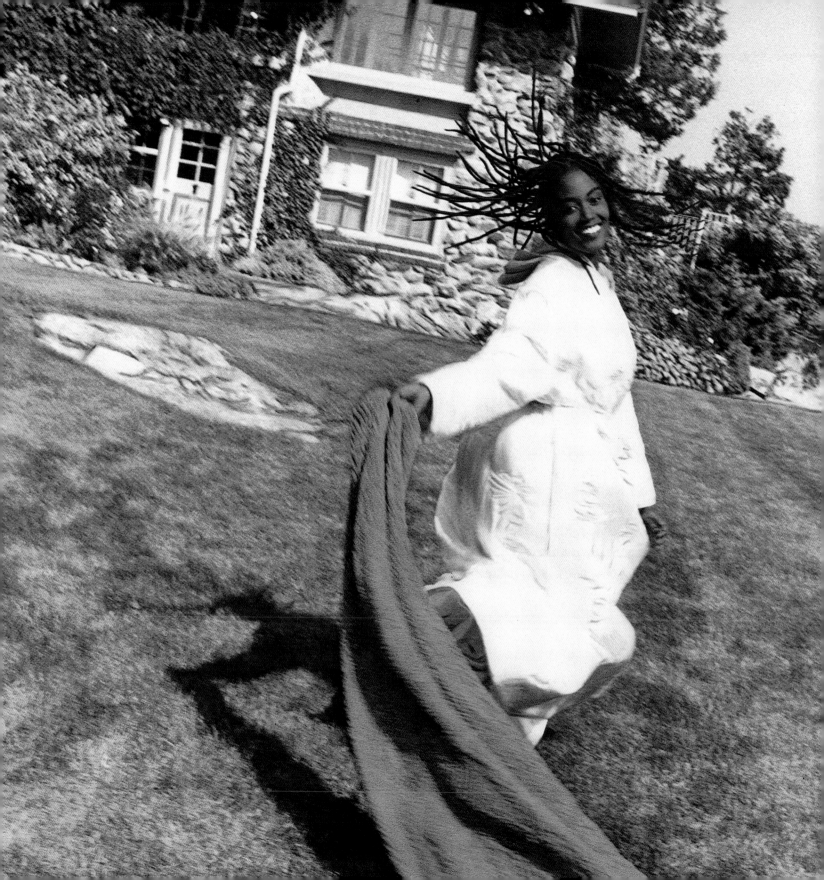

love interest—in that spoken-word poetry class we've been threatening to take. Great minds think alike. Have faith that in time God places the right people in our lives.

Resolving Conflict

Let's be honest. Sometimes the people in our lives get on our last nerve. Maybe it's a younger sister, who has the annoying habit of getting along with our parents better than we

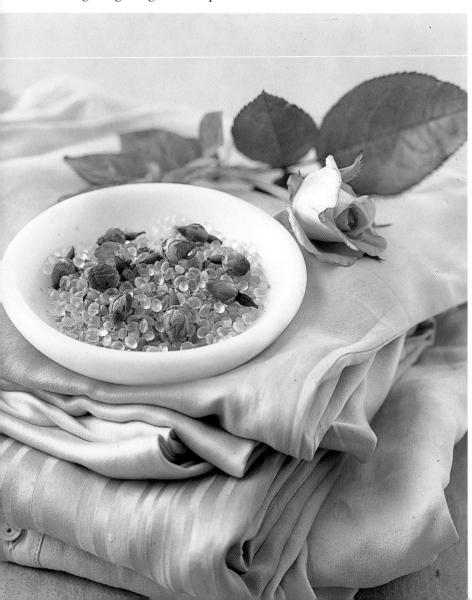

Aroma beads release soothing fragrances.

do. Perhaps it's the friend whose company we love but who is perpetually late to everything. We're talking silly, petty irritations that reflect more on us than they do on the person who's gotten under our skin. Can we just let it go? If the answer is no because it seems to hang on no matter what we do, we need to think long and hard about what's really bothering us. We may need to talk to the person with whom we feel conflict or drop them a note. We have to be honest and ask ourselves: "Is there any part I'm playing in the conflict?" Or, if we've done the soul searching and discovered that it really is *our* problem, we may need to bend the ear of a wise friend to get a new perspective on it all. The point is for us to be free of anything that might clip our wings.

Getting Centered

Have you ever noticed that when you're anxious, your breathing becomes shallow? If you're around your mama, what's the first thing she says? Take a deep breath, girl, and try to calm down. Shallow breaths come from the chest, deep breaths from the diaphragm. In just a few minutes of breathing from your center, you can restore your composure.

We have a spiritual center that is the counterpart of our physical one. When we're "centered," we feel tranquillity. People and circumstances move around us without throwing us off balance. Even in times of crisis, we know the storm will pass.

One way we can enhance our sense of being centered is to spend time in nature. If you live in an urban area, find your way to a park. In nature, every tree, every animal, every blade of grass is in its divine right place. So are you. Can you feel it?

Joy is a natural expression of knowing God. If you tend to be critical and/or to see everything that's wrong in a situation, begin to shift your thinking. We should find the good in the world and praise it. Pay attention to the ratio of positive-to-negative comments that you make. Each day, find something to admire about the people you work and/or live with, and tell them about it. When you approach the world with a smile, people feel you, doors open, you create your own good luck.

But it's not all about you. If you see a friend or family member who appears to be a quart low in spirit, be willing to put your program on hold long enough so you can share an inspirational passage with them or pray that the circumstances weighing them down will lift from their shoulders. Consider that your well-lived life may be an example to others. Perhaps you have an idea for an after-school program or a community resource center. Who's to say you can't start one? On a smaller, but equally meaningful scale, think about volunteering; teaching someone to read, sponsoring a Little League softball team. We often underestimate how much a little effort on our parts might light up someone else's life.

IYANLA VANZANT'S INTERNAL BEAUTY REGIMEN

Once upon a time there was a little girl so convinced that she was ugly that she spent hours staring into the mirror, praying to be transformed into a beauty. One day, as she gazed at her reflection, she saw a woman dressed in flowing white robes, glowing with a radiant beauty beyond belief. The future Iyanla Vanzant extended her hand and told the young girl, "All your beauty is within. It is your power."

It took the girl years to realize that the gorgeous woman speaking such soothing words of wisdom was the grown-up version of herself, her spirit reaching out to comfort her across space and time. Today, Iyanla Vanzant understands that the body is an extension of the soul, and that finding the beauty within is the key to spiritual well-being.

"You can't really separate spiritual and mental well-being," says Vanzant, an award-winning author, minister, lawyer, and spiritual counselor. "One of the best ways we can achieve spiritual well-being is to praise everything. Praise is the greatest way to bring yourself into the presence of God. Ask the Holy Spirit to show you the love in every situation."

To find your own inner beauty, Vanzant suggests the following eight steps to keep your mind, body, and soul in perfect harmony:

1. **Know the truth: We are all connected to the omnipotent, omnipresence called the Creator.**

2. **Be grateful for everything.**

3. **Develop and maintain an individual and intimate relationship with the God of your understanding.**

4. **Learn to be involved with yourself so that you can evolve in the world.**

5. **Learn the difference between thinking and consciousness. Thinking is a function of the external world and we respond to the stimuli from outside sources. Consciousness is a process of unfolding through acknowledgment and acceptance of your own internal divinity.**

6. **Know and live your principles.**

7. **Replace want with desire. Wanting is a mental construct that acknowledges that something is lacking. Desire is an internal acknowledgment of what already exists.**

8. **Replace need with creation. Need is also a mental construct based on physical stimulation. Creation is the utilization of your true nature, which is divine. We can create whatever we want to experience.**

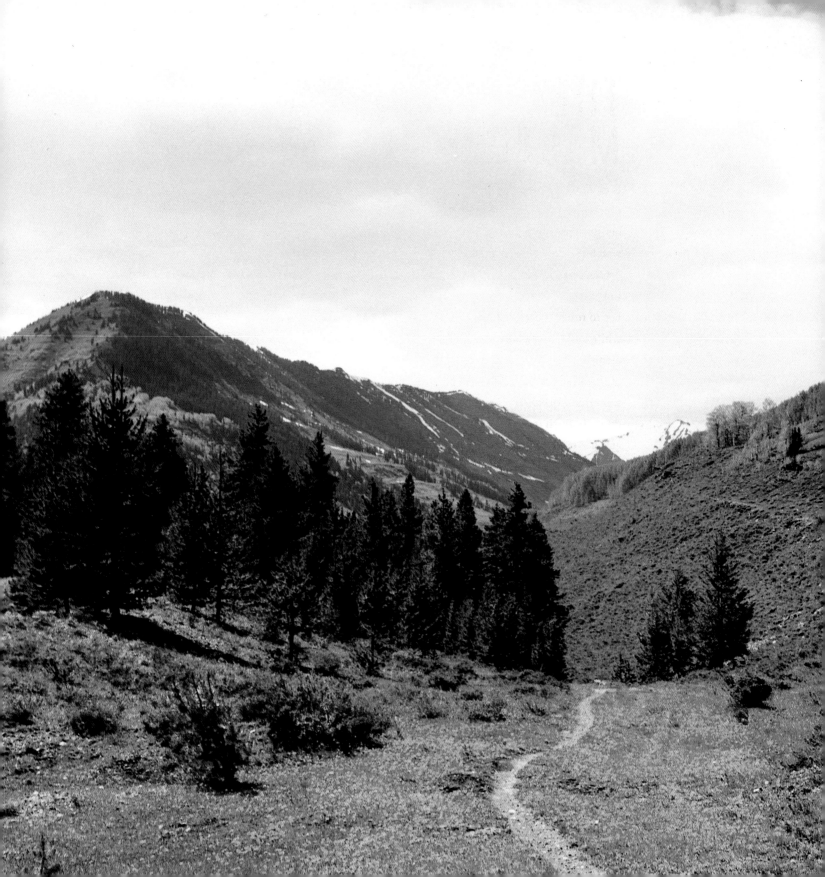

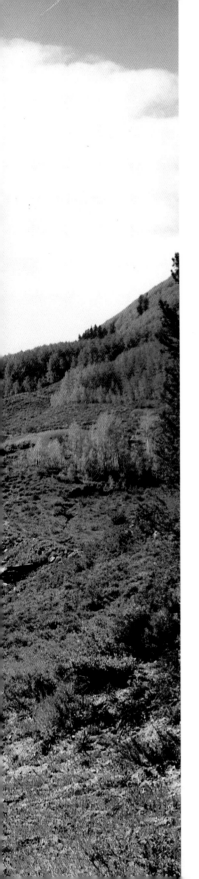

THE MAKEOVER

Putting in long hours on the job made Carol a professional superstar, but the toll it took on her personal life made her wonder if it was all worth it.

Carol was running on fumes. Her demanding career as an advertising executive pressed her to reach higher and higher sales goals, while at the same time managing a staff of fifteen. If a business meeting didn't pull her out of the office for lunch, she would often grab something quick, like fried chicken or hot dogs. To burn it off, she preferred swimming at a health club near her home. But many nights she was too exhausted to even stop at the club, and instead headed home and straight to bed. On top of it all, she was a half-pack-a-day smoker, a habit she wanted to kick but couldn't seem to.

Overwhelmed by stress, Carol's spirit was crying out for a total mind-body makeover. *Essence* heard her plea and sent her to the New Age Health Spa Lifestyles Program in Neversink, New York.

Spas like the one Carol went to are not designed simply to give you a few days of bliss before sending you back into battle. The concept is to offer you new, mindful ways to manage the pressures in your everyday life.

By combining Western medical practices with Asian and other nontraditional treatment systems, the spa staff helped Carol get her groove back and realize that she *was* in control of her life.

Getting Going

At the spa, Carol met individually with the medical director, as well as experts in psychoanalysis, physical fitness, nutrition, and emerging fields such as acupuncture and health kinesiology to establish where she was in her life and where she wanted to go.

Rob, the spa nutritionist, introduced Carol to some new ways of thinking about eating. During a special meditation, Rob asked Carol to visualize the steps grapes might take from growing in a vineyard to arriving as a box of raisins in the pantry at home. Slowing down and learning to appreciate the taste and complexity of food helped her better gauge her appetite, avoid overeating, and enjoy her meals more. Because *how* we eat is as important as *what* we eat, Rob suggested Carol consider "mindful" eating as part of an overall philosophy of mindful living. He encouraged her to share her emotions and feelings, dealing with them in the present rather than choking them down by overeating.

Menu Makeover

Together, Rob and Carol devised a plan for her to eat three to five small meals a day. Much of the food in the plan was not only nutritious but also quick and easy to prepare—something especially important to high-powered women like Carol. Cereal, fruit, and whole-grain breads were her morning options, while fresh salads were recommended when she dined out with business clients or even grabbed something on the go. For meals at home, the spa chef taught Carol a few time-saving culinary tricks to make preparing tasty soups and salads fast and fun.

Arleen, the spa's fitness instructor, also had some valuable advice for Carol. Her "intake inventory" showed that though Carol some-times walked after work for exercise, she wasn't getting enough health benefit from her efforts. Taking into consideration where Carol lived, Arleen designed a simple routine for Carol to briskly walk to the park ten minutes from her home, alternately walk and jog while at the park, and then stretch and stride home.

For her next treatment, Carol tried acupunc-ture. Dr. Renu Jerath used this ancient Chinese medical technique to tap Carol's six meridians, or energy channels. By painlessly sticking tiny needles in her "trigger points," Dr. Jerath helped alleviate some of Carol's health concerns. A set of needles placed in her back for a few minutes, for instance, eased the pain she was feeling in her neck, shoulders, and upper back. Dr. Jerath also left a group of minute pins in Carol's ears for several days to boost her energy and reduce her urge to smoke. Whenever she felt a need to light up, all Carol had to do was gently rub the tacks in her ear and many times her urge for a smoke went away.

Upping the Energy

Jo-Ann, the spa's health kinesiologist, worked with Carol using a number of techniques, including "chelation" therapy. Jo-Ann explained that with chelation therapy, also based on Chinese principles of energy and flow, she drew energy up from the earth and passed it on to Carol's body. The idea being that by channeling energy in this way, Carol's body would choose where it needed attention most. Like a detective sifting through evi-dence, Jo-Ann moved her hands an inch or two away from the surface of Carol's skin, starting at her feet and moving upwards until she felt the energy blockage at the throat chakra (one of seven energy centers in the body). It was there that the barrier to energy flow was so great that Carol felt an intense heat in and around her neck. Jo-Ann gave her flower essences—like those used in aro-matherapy oils—designed to reconnect the body's electrical system and get the energy circulating again. However, the deeper mes-sage Carol's throat chakra was sending her would only be realized later.

Mindful Meditation

Some of the most important ground Carol cov-ered at the spa was with Bernice, a psychother-

Opposite: The power of prayer is wondrous.

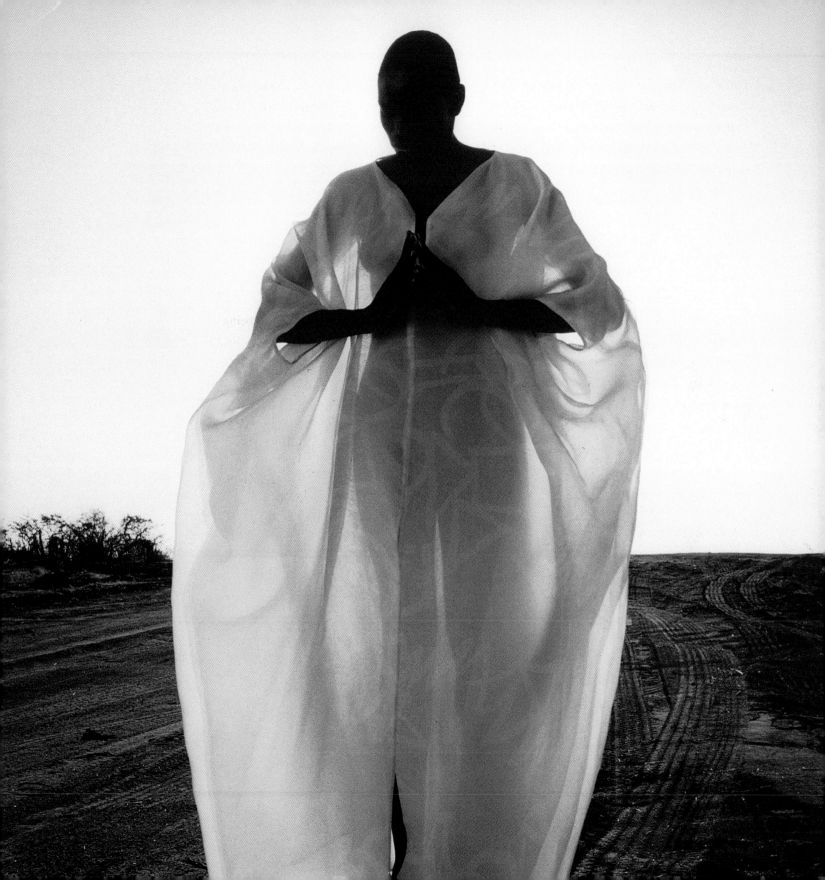

apist. The two met at least twice a day over the course of the week they worked together, and it was during these one-on-one sessions that several important things about Carol's life came to light.

Much of Bernice's work was based on establishing the connection between the body and the mind. She called it "uncovering the thumbtack," because many times the source of our mental and spiritual discomfort is only a small memory, experience, or situation from the past buried beneath layers of time. These thumbtacks are either in our minds or our hearts, Bernice said, and until we dig deep and find them, it is difficult to heal ourselves. It's like taking aspirin without finding out what's causing the pain in the first place.

For example, Carol frequently fell asleep during "mindful meditation" sessions. Instead of inner peace, Bernice suggested that Carol's tiredness was a mental and spiritual fatigue stemming from her unconscious desire to escape or avoid confronting a deep-rooted concern or problem. This observation rang true when Carol was suddenly overcome by an unexplainable sadness and began to cry during one particular meeting early in the week. This was a surprise for both women, but especially for Carol herself, because she insisted that she rarely cried—and never when other people were around.

During each daily session, Bernice encouraged Carol to look for the source of her sad-ness. As they talked about her life, Bernice noted that Carol was torn in the relationships she had with her parents, who had divorced years before. She felt very close to her mother, and respected her for being a self-assured, upbeat woman. Yet when she filled out a questionnaire at the first session with Bernice, Carol's responses included her sense that "people are inherently self-protective and defensive." Such thoughts and feelings pointed to a cynical perspective that could have been influenced by her father's own pessimistic outlook.

Finding Her Voice

The big breakthrough occurred when Bernice established a link between Carol's life and that of her mother. Carol's mother was forty-eight years old when she divorced Carol's father and began an almost entirely new life filled with the things she had always wanted to do. The significance of her mother's new lifestyle was not lost on Carol, who, coincidentally, was forty-eight when she visited the spa.

Bernice helped Carol to see that she did not have to "own" the negativity from the past. The important thing for her to do instead was to search for creative expression and do the "things" she wanted to do in life. Take piano lessons. Mentor young people. Study modern dance. Carol had already found a "voice" in the career world. But Bernice told her that the sadness in her heart—that lump in her throat—would only disappear when she reconnected with her personal life and found a creative voice for self-expression.

It was after these sessions that everything she'd learned at the spa crystallized for Carol. Before the visit, her life had felt like a one-way dead-end street. Though the business lunches, the travel opportunities, and the high-profile projects made her job seem glamorous, she would get so tied up in the busyness of business that she hardly had any energy left to pursue her own personal dreams. So while it was relaxing to spend a week getting away from it all, the true test for Carol was returning to the real world.

Bringing It On Home

Some of the lifestyle changes she made at the spa were easy to keep. She stuck to the eating plan instead of stuffing herself with fast food. By eating mindfully, she found that she liked the variety found in salads, and she ordered them more often when dining out. At home, her new cooking skills came in handy when preparing satisfying exotic dishes like wild rice crepes with seasonal vegetables or carrot ginger soup.

At the spa, Carol was reminded of how good it felt to exercise regularly. To stay active, she made plans to start swimming again—this time with a friend from the office, so they could encourage each other. Though she found it challenging to exercise full-time, when she did work out in the park, she knew how to maximize her time by training effectively with a quick pace.

Giving up cigarettes, however, still proved a struggle. Although her goal was to quit completely, she was encouraged when she found herself smoking half as much as she did before her trip to the spa. After Dr. Jerath, Jo-Ann, and Bernice used completely different practices and came up with similar results— whether a need to find a voice, shoulder and neck pain, or an energy blockage at the throat chakra—Carol began to see those "nicotine sticks" as a symbol for all the negative things she was doing to block the flow of her life. With a newfound awareness of her mind-body connection, she began to think before she lit up, and to tell herself, sometimes, that she really didn't want or need a cigarette at that moment.

Carol also set about finding a voice in her personal life. She followed up on her sessions with Bernice and began looking for a music teacher and spent a few Saturday afternoons window shopping for a piano keyboard. And remembering the positive influences elders had on her life, she volunteered at a local high school to teach life and career skills to at-risk teenage girls.

Her time at the spa helped Carol to see that she had been leading an unbalanced life. But like her mother, who was forty-eight years young when she changed her life for the better, Carol, at the same age, stepped out in a new, rewarding direction.

RESOURCE LIST CONSULTANTS FOR *THE ESSENCE TOTAL MAKEOVER*

MAKEOVER CONSULTANTS

Skin

Irma Denson
Irma Denson Skin Care Salon
  and Day Spa
155 East 55th Street
New York, NY 10022
(212) 371-3413

Dr. Deborah A. Simmons
132 West 96th Street
New York, NY 10025
(212) 865-3376

Hair

Diane Dacosta
Dyaspora Hair Salon & Day Spa
37 West End Avenue
New York, NY 10023
(212) 265-9292

Diane Bailey
Tendrils House of Ujamma
154 Vanderbilt Avenue
Brooklyn, NY 11205
(718) 875-3811

George Buckner
Hair Fashions East
411 Park Avenue South
New York, NY 10016
(212) 686-7524

Ellin LaVar
LaVar Hair Designs
127 West 72nd Street
New York, NY 10023
(212) 724-4492

Body

Ryan Gentles
Zion Physical Wellness
Cooper Station
PO Box 1392
New York, NY 10276
(917) 894-4646

Sharone Huey
New York Sports Training
  Institute
575 Lexington Avenue
New York, NY 10022
(212) 752-7111

Nutrition

Constance Brown-Riggs, M.S.Ed.,
  R.D., C.D.E., C.D.N.
5724 Merrick Road
Massapequa, NY 11758
(516) 795-4288

Mental Wellness

Linda Anderson, Ph.D.
170 West 73rd Street
New York, NY 10023
(212) 595-7302

Beatrice Brown, Ph.D.
BSB Wholistic Health Center
689 Locust Street
Mount Vernon, NY 10552
(914) 699-1615

Spiritual Wellness

Werner Mendel
New Age Health Spa
Route 55
Neversink, NY 12765
(914) 985-7601

MAKEOVER FITNESS CENTERS

New York Health & Racquet
  Club
24 East 13th Street
New York, NY 10003
(212) 924-4600

New York Sports Training
  Institute
575 Lexington Avenue
New York, NY 10022
(212) 752-7111

Revolution Studios
104 East 14th Street
New York, NY 10003
(212) 206-8785

SPAS

Spa Hotline (800) ALL-SPAS or
(212) 924-6800
Spa Trek (800) 272-3480 or
(212) 779-3480

Spa Atlantis (resort)
Pompano Beach, Florida
(800) 583-3500

Green Mountain at Fox Run
  (weight loss)
Ludlow, Vermont
(800) 448-8106

Harbour Village Beach Resort
  (resort)
Bonaire, Dutch Caribbean
(800) 424-0004

Jackie's on the Reef
  (destination)
Negril, Jamaica
(718) 469-2785 (reservations)
(876) 957-4997 (Jamaica)

Lake Austin Spa Resort
  (destination)
Austin, Texas
(800) 847-5637

The Oaks At Ojai (destination)
Ojai, California
(805) 646-5573

INFORMATION HOTLINES

New Age Health Spa (health)
Neversink, New York
(800) 682-4348

New Life Fitness Vacations
   (resort)
Killington, Vermont
(800) 545-9407

Sanibel Harbor Resort and Spa
   (resort)
Fort Myers, Florida
(800) 767-7777

Sans Souci Lido (resort)
Ocho Rios, Jamaica
(876) 974-2353

Structure House (weight loss)
Durham, North Carolina
(800) 553-0052

Tennessee Fitness Spa
   (destination)
Waynesboro, Tennessee
(931) 722-5589

Wildwood Lifestyle Center and
   Hospital (health)
Wildwood, Georgia
(800) 634-9355

ALCOHOLICS ANONYMOUS (212) 870-3400 or check your local listings.

AMERICAN ANOREXIA AND BULIMIA ASSOCIATION (212) 575-6200 or check your local listings.

AMERICAN CANCER SOCIETY (212) 586-8700

AMERICAN MASSAGE THERAPY ASSOCIATION (847) 864-0123

CANCER INFORMATION SERVICE—NATIONAL CANCER INSTITUTE (800) 4-CANCER

CONSUMER CREDIT COUNSELING SERVICES (800) 388-2227 or (800) 547-5005

CRISIS INTERVENTION HOTLINE (800) 866-9600 or check your local listings.

DEBTORS ANONYMOUS (781) 453-2743

DOMESTIC VIOLENCE HOTLINE (800) 621-4673

GAMBLERS ANONYMOUS (212) 903-4400

HERB RESEARCH FOUNDATION (303) 449-2265

MEDICAL LIBRARY: THE NEW YORK ACADEMY OF MEDICINE (212) 822-7327

NARCOTICS ANONYMOUS (212) 929-6262 or check your local listings.

NATIONAL CENTER FOR HEALTH STATISTICS (301) 436-8500

NATIONAL HIV AND AIDS HOTLINE (800) 342-2437

NATIONAL INSTITUTES OF HEALTH (301) 402-1770

NATIONAL LIBRARY OF MEDICINE (301) 496-1030. Reference: (888) FIND NLM x2

NATIONAL MEDICAL ASSOCIATION (202) 347-1895

OVEREATERS ANONYMOUS (505) 891-2664

SMOKENDERS (800) 828-4357

ACKNOWLEDGMENTS

This book would not have been possible without the great generosity of the photographers and the dedication of the *Essence* team.

Organizing a timeless makeover book is a formidable task, and it is most rewarding to have accomplished it with the tireless efforts of the talented and committed Essence Books staff: Zurn Porter, my trusted assistant; Knox Robinson, assistant editor; Tracy Harford, photo editor and books assistant; and Carol Banks, books assistant. Special thanks to the *Essence* art department for their invaluable help: LaVon Leak-Wilks, Jan DeChabert, Fabienne Dougé, Lauri Lyons, Leah Rudolpho, and Rob Vano.

Special thanks to the *Essence* family for their collaborated efforts: Sandra Martin for her tremendous assistance and support, and to Derryale Barnes, Janice K. Bryant, Ayana M. Davis, Sherrill Clarke, Elayne Fluker, Ziba Kashef, Marsha Kelly, Yvette Russell, and Taiia Smart-Young. Many thanks to Akissi Britton, Annetta McKenzie, Debra Parker, Constance Reid, Christine Reisner, Wilma Remy, and Rashida Wright. We are grateful to Amiyr Barclift, Arcadia Caraballo, Adriane Carter, Natalee Huey, Audrey Adams-Maillian, Larry Ramo, Jackie Richardson, Annette Simmons, Robert Vopelak, and Denise West. Much appreciation to Greg Boyea and Edgerton Maloney, as well as Amanda Cadogan, Denolyn Carol, Trudi Hewitt, Kathryn Daniels, Ihsan Muhammad, and Janice Wheeler.

Many thanks to our designer Elizabeth Van Itallie, to our makeover photographers Deborah Feingold and Charles Pizzarello, and to our makeover participants: Victoria Brown, Lisa Christmas, Natalie Cosby, Carol Cunningham, Stephanie Dash, Natasha Gray, Michele Griffin, Belinda Holmes, Tareeka Kelly, Tracie Morrison, Joyce Pounds, LaShena Verrett, and our mental and spiritual wellness participants.

Additional thanks to those who provided our writers with their expertise: Nadia Abdur-Rahman; Queen Afua, Heal Thyself Center, New York; Sandi Allen; Olive Benson, Olive's Hair Salon, Boston; Lorenza Bailey; Julia Boyd; Dr. Denise Buntin; Denise Cavassa; Dr. William Coffey; Dr. Andi Coleman; Dr. Fran Cook-Bolden; Crystal Devin, Crystal's Royal Secrets, New York; Jewel Diamond Taylor; Robin Emtage; Sam Fine; Dr. Ophelia Finley Oliver; Barry Fletcher, Avant Garde Hair Gallery, Capital Heights; Anita Gibson; Gwendolyn Goldsby Grant, Ed.D.; Grandmaster Asar Ha-Pi, Ph.D., A New Horizon Health Services, Chicago; Theresa Harmon; Kennise Herring; Debrena Jackson-Gandy, Masterminds, Seattle; Clayton James; Victoria Johnson; Dr. William Keith; Marcia Kilgore; Dr. Lewanzer Lassiter; Lanier Long; Kevin Martin; Jean Miller, Ph.D., BodyCentered, New York; Dr. Denise Shirvington; Andrea Sullivan; Dr. Ella Toombs; Iyanla Vanzant; Brenda Wade, Ph.D., Heartline Productions, San Francisco; Rob Willis, Rob Willis International, Southfield; Jae Wilson.

An abundance of gratitude to Edward Lewis, Clarence O. Smith, Susan L. Taylor, Harry Dedyo, Elaine P. Williams, Jim Forsythe, Bill Knight, and Barbara Britton.

At Crown, special appreciation to Steve Ross, Ayesha Pande, and Lauren Dong.

PHOTOGRAPHY CREDITS

Page 2: David Sacks
7: Charlie Pizzarello
11: Brad Hitz

LOVING OUR SKIN

Page 12: Didier Gault
14 top: Mark Havriliak
14 bottom left, center, right:
    Matthew Jordan Smith
15: Charlie Pizzarello
16: Idaljiza Liz-Lepiorz
17: Michael Myers
18: Charlie Pizzarello
19: Johnathan Kantor
20: Bruno Gaget
21: Matthew Jordan Smith
22: Paul Lange
23: Kip Meyer
24: Matthew Jordan Smith
25: Troy Word
26: Paul Lange
29: Matthew Jordan Smith
30: Matthew Jordan Smith
33: Bruno Gaget
34: Didier Gault
35: Carlton Davis
36: Matthew Jordan Smith
37: Bruno Gaget
38: David Roth
39: Francesco Mosto
40: Charlie Pizzarello
41 top: Michael Lisnet
41 bottom: Bruno Gaget
42 top left: Matthew Jordan Smith
42 top right and bottom:
    Francesco Mosto
43: Charlie Pizzarello
44–45: John Peden
46 left: Didier Gault
46 right: Matthew Jordan Smith
47 left: Matthew Jordan Smith
47 right: Mark Havriliak
48: Warren Mantooth

49: Ronnie Wright
    (courtesy of Arista Records)
50: Charlie Pizzarello
51: Deborah Feingold
52: Charlie Pizzarello
53: Deborah Feingold
54: Charlie Pizzarello
55: Deborah Feingold

CELEBRATING OUR HAIR

Page 56: Matthew Jordan Smith
58 left: Charlie Pizzarello
58 center: Mark Havriliak
58 right: Keith Major
59: Matthew Jordan Smith
60–61: Charlie Pizzarello
62: Barron Claiborne
63: Matthew Jordan Smith
64: Paul Lange
65: Antoine Bootz
66: Matthew Jordan Smith
67: John Peden
68: John Peden
69: Charles Bush (courtesy of
    Columbia Records)
70: Matthew Jordan Smith
71: Francesco Mosto
72: Bruno Gaget
73: Didier Gault
74–75: Matthew Jordan Smith
76 top left: Charlie Pizzarello
76 bottom right: Michael Myers
77: Marc Baptiste
78: Dennis Mitchell
81: Dennis Mitchell
82–83: Matthew Jordan Smith
84: Davis Factor
86 top: Charlie Pizzarello
86 bottom: Deborah Feingold
87 top: Charlie Pizzarello
87 bottom: Deborah Feingold
88: Charlie Pizzarello
89: Deborah Feingold

90 top: Charlie Pizzarello
90 bottom: Deborah Feingold
91 top: Deborah Feingold
91 bottom: Charlie Pizzarello

BODY BEAUTIFUL

Page 92: Barron Claiborne
94: Matthew Jordan Smith
95: Kip Meyer
96: Adrian Buckmaster
97: Marc Baptiste
99: Matthew Jordan Smith
100: Matthew Jordan Smith
101: Kip Meyer
102: Frits Berends
103: Timothy Hill
104: Matthew Jordan Smith
105: Warren Mantooth
106: Stephen Churchill Downes
107: Paul B. Goode
108: Nick Vaccaro
109: Charlie Pizzarello
110: Idaljiza Liz-Lepiorz
112–113: Mark Seelen
115: Charlie Pizzarello
116: Mark Havriliak
117 left: Carlton Davis
117 right: Bruno Gaget
119: Idaljiza Liz-Lepiorz
120: Michael Myers
122: Charlie Pizzarello
123: Deborah Feingold
124: Charlie Pizzarello
125: Deborah Feingold

HEALTHY LIVING

Page 126: Rita Maas
128: Rita Maas
129: Charlie Pizzarello
130: Stephen Mark Needham
131: Rita Maas
132: Kip Meyer
133: Rita Maas
135 top: Cynthia Brown

135 bottom: Rick Osentoski
136: James Sorenson
137: Rita Maas
140–141: Charlie Pizzarello
142: Charlie Pizzarello
144: David Sacks
148: Idaljiza Liz-Lepiorz
153: Idaljiza Liz-Lepiorz
156: Charlie Pizzarello
157: Deborah Feingold
158: Charlie Pizzarello
159: Deborah Feingold

MENTAL WELLNESS

Page 160: Carl Posey
163: Ruven Afanador
164: Benoit Malphettes
166: Ellen Silverman
167: Frits Berends
170: Warren Mantooth
171: Idaljiza Liz-Lepiorz
172: Ruven Afanador
176–177: Joanne Chan
178–179: Kip Meyer
180–181: Ellen Silverman
182: Marc Baptiste

SPIRITUAL POWER

Page 184: Anthony Barboza
186: Frits Berends
188: Charlie Pizzarello
189: Frits Berends
191: Ruven Afanador
192: Marc Baptiste
193: Idaljiza Liz-Lepiorz
195: William Richards
197: Ruven Afanador
198: Frits Berends
199: Ellen Silverman
201: Idaljiza Liz-Lepiorz
202: Ellen Silverman
204–205: Warren Mantooth
207: Marc Baptiste

INDEX

faith, 189–90

feet, 109–10, 112–14, 118

fibroids, 147

finasteride, 80

flesh moles, 31

Fletcher, Barry, 85

folate, 136, 139, 148

food. *See* diet and nutrition

forgiveness, 193–95

foundation (makeup), 41

G

Gentles, Ryan, 154, 155, 157–59

Giovanni, Nikki, 151

gratitude, 195

grief, 168–70

H

hair, 57–91

    alopecia, 74, 79–80, 87

    basic care tools, 70–71

    braids and natural looks, 76–77, 79, 87

    breakage of, 80, 85

    coloring of, 62, 68, 79, 82–85

    condition assessment, 61–62

    conditioning of, 68–71, 73, 76, 77, 79, 82, 85

    dandruff, 54, 67, 80

    eyebrows, 44–45

    facial, 28, 31, 32, 50

    locks, 77–79

    makeover stories, 86–91

    relaxers, 54, 62, 68, 73, 79

    shampooing of, 54, 66–68, 73, 76–77, 79

    shaving of, 31, 50, 111

structure of, 62–66

stylist selection, 81

waxing of, 28, 45, 50, 114

weaves, 74, 76, 79, 87

hands, 110–11, 112

Ha-Pi, Asar, 106

health and fitness, 93–159

    alternative healing, 144–45

    basic body care, 108–13

    makeover stories, 122–25, 154–59

    medical issues, 130, 139–43, 146–54

    posture, 95

    problems and remedies, 120–21

    self-assessment of, 94, 128

    special treatments, 114–19

    See also diet and nutrition; exercise; mental wellness

heart disease, 150–51, 152

herbs, 85, 144–45

Hill, Lauryn, 192–93

HIV, 151–52

hives, 33

hormone replacement therapy, 150

Horne, Lena, 140

hot combs, 85

hotlines, information, 211

Huey, Sharone, 107, 122–24

hydroquinone, 32

hyperpigmentation, 32

hypertension, 150–52

hysterectomy, 147

I

immune system, 79, 146

inner peace, 199–203

intuition, 200

J

Jackson, Janet, 111

Jerath, Dr. Renu, 206, 209

Johnson, Dr. Beverly (dermatologist), 36

Johnson, Beverly (model), 45

Jordan, Patrice, 24–25

Joyner-Kersee, Jackie, 140

K

Keith, Dr. William D., 36

keloids, 32, 108

kickboxing, 103

L

laser surgery, 31, 35–36, 121

Lassiter, Dr. Lewanzer, 154

LaVar, Ellin, 86

legs, 100–101, 108–9, 111, 121

Lewis, Jackie, 194

liposuction, 120

lips, 20, 38, 45, 48

locks, 77–79

Long, Lanier, 48

Long, Nia, 20

loss, coping with, 162, 168–70

love, 190, 193

lupus, 146, 151

M

Mackey, Kendra, 101

makeup, 28, 38–49

    basic tools, 38–39

    camera and photography tips, 47–48

    for eyes, 38, 41–48

for lips, 45, 48

mistake remedies, 47–48

powders and foundations, 41–42, 47

removal of, 16–18

special looks, 46–47, 48

manic depression, 178

manicures, 110–11, 112

mascara, 42, 44, 48

mask of pregnancy, 32

masks, skin care, 24, 119

massage, 23, 114, 117

McKinley-Grant, Dr. Lynn, 36

meditation, 27, 193, 196–99

menopause, 32, 79, 148–50

menstruation, 27, 147–48

mental wellness, 161–83

    addiction, 174

    depression, 165, 166, 168

    eating disorders, 175

    loss issues, 168–70

    makeover stories, 180–83

    manic depression, 178

    money concerns, 175–77

    moodiness, 165–66

    relationship issues, 170–74

    self-assessment of, 162

    therapist selection, 179

    See also spirituality

Miller, Dr. Carlyle H., 154

minerals, 138, 139

minoxidil, 80

moisturizers

    hair, 67, 68, 73, 77, 82

    skin, 16, 18–20, 27, 28, 32, 36, 109–10

moles, 31, 32, 33

money issues, 162, 175–77

Monica, 49

moodiness, 165–66, 178

Morrison, Toni, 166